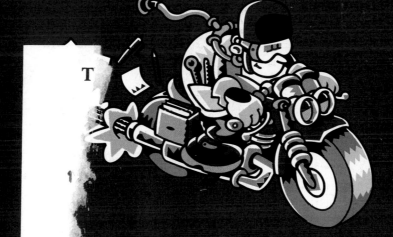

Cell Biology and Genetics

Series editor
Daniel Horton-Szar
BSc (Hons)
United Medical and Dental
Schools of Guy's and
St Thomas's Hospitals
(UMDS),
London

Faculty advisor
Michael C. Steel
MBChB, PhD, DSc, FRCPE,
FRCSE, FRCPath, FRSE
Professor in Medical Science
University of St Andrews
Fife

Cell Biology and Genetics

Emma C.A. Jones
BSc (Hons)
United Medical and
Dental Schools of Guy's
and St Thomas's
Hospitals (UMDS),
London

Anna Morris
BSc (Hons)
United Medical and
Dental Schools of Guy's
and St Thomas's
Hospitals (UMDS),
London

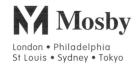 Mosby

London • Philadelphia
St Louis • Sydney • Tokyo

Editor	**Louise Crowe**
Development Editors	**Filipa Maia**
	Michelle Campbell
Project Manager	**Cathryn Waters**
Designer	**Greg Smith**
Layout	**Gisli Thor**
Illustration Management	**Danny Pyne**
Illustrators	**Mick Ruddy**
	Mike Saiz
	Milvia Romici
	Sandie Hill
Cover Design	**Greg Smith**
Production	**Siobhan Egan**
Index	**Liza Weinkove**

ISBN 0 7234 3135 3

Copyright © Mosby International Ltd, 1998.

Published by Mosby, an imprint of Mosby International Ltd, Lynton House, 7–12 Tavistock Square, London WC1H 9LB, UK.

Printed in Barcelona, Spain, by Grafos S.A. Arte sobre papel, 1998.
Text set in Crash Course–VAG Light; captions in Crash Course–VAG Thin.

Cataloguing in Publication Data
Catalogue records for this book are available from the British Library and the US Library of Congress.

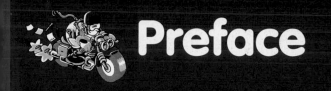

Preface

This book brings together the basic concepts of cell biology and molecular genetics that the medical student is required to know. The style of the text is concise and to the point, with many illustrations to make this book approachable and easy to understand. A good understanding of cell biology is essential, not only to pass exams, but also to understand molecular techniques including gene tracking and gene therapy, techniques that are becoming an integral part of all fields of medicine.

The text has been based around our pre-clinical and genetics degree lecture notes, which were formed when studying in the excellent molecular biology and genetics departments at Guy's and St Thomas's. The more important concepts have been highlighted, and illustrations have been used, where possible, to explain concepts where text often fails. This book is extensive but, we hope, simple to master.

Emma C. A. Jones
Anna Morris

Integration of the concepts of basic science into clinical practice is an ambitious but necessary goal for medical teaching in the 21st century. This volume reflects that objective, allowing the student at the very start of the course to look ahead to the clinical relevance of cell structure, biochemical pathways and the principles of Mendelian genetics. Equally, those students with more experience of 'real live' patients can remind themselves of the scientific foundations on which diagnosis and treatment rest.

Although a great deal of information has been compressed into relatively few pages, care has been taken to restate important scientific concepts, in the later chapters, in their clinical contexts, so that each section of the text is self-supporting and readable.

Any student who has mastered the material contained in this slim volume should have little to fear from the examiners, but the objective is not simply to help you over these hurdles. The authors and editors would hope that the book may serve as a quick reference guide for students and qualified doctors alike as they encounter problems in the wide field of genetics, and that some, at least, may be encouraged to develop a special interest in this challenging area of medicine.

Professor Michael C. Steel
Faculty Advisor

Preface

OK, no-one ever said medicine was going to be easy, but the thing is, there are very few parts of this enormous subject that are actually difficult to understand. The problem for most of us is the sheer volume of information that must be absorbed before each round of exams. It's not fun when time is getting short and you realize that: (a) you really should have done a bit more work by now and (b) there are large gaps in your lecture notes that you meant to copy up but never quite got round to.

This series has been designed and written by senior medical students and doctors with recent experience of basic medical science exams. We've brought together all the information you need into compact, manageable volumes that integrate basic science with clinical skills. There is a consistent structure and layout across the series, and every title is checked for accuracy by senior faculty members from medical schools across the UK.

I hope this book makes things a little easier!

Danny Horton-Szar
Series Editor (Basic Medical Sciences)

Acknowledgements

A special thanks to my father, Dr J. H. Morris, whose support helped make this book possible for me. Anna Morris.

Figure Credits

Figures 1.1, 2.3, 4.5, 4.6A, 4.7, 4.9, 4.12–4.15, 4.28, 5.2–4, 5.6 & 6.10 adapted from *Human Histology 2e,* by Dr A. Stevens and Professor J. Lowe, Mosby 1997.

Figure 5.3, redrawn from an electromicrograph, taken from *Human Histology 2e,* by Dr A. Stevens and Professor J. Lowe, Mosby 1997.

Figure 2.15 adapted from *Clinical Chemistry 3e,* by Dr W. J. Marshall, Mosby, 1995.

Figure 5.20 adapted from *Medical Genetics,* by Dr L.B. Jorde, Dr J.C. Carey and Dr R. L. White, Mosby Year Book, 1997.

Contents

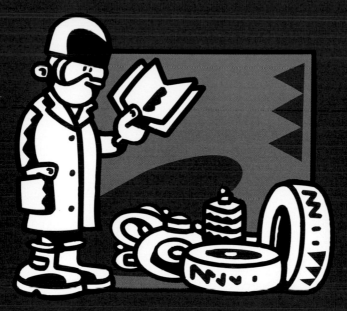

PRINCIPLES OF CELL BIOLOGY AND MOLECULAR GENETICS

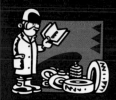

1. General Organization of the Cell

CELL CONCEPT

Introduction

The word 'cell' was first used by Robert Hooke in 1665 when he observed that cork viewed under the microscope was composed of numerous similar structures. The cell theory, proposed by Schleiden and Schwann in 1839, states that cells are of universal occurrence and are the basic units of an organism. In 1855 Virchow restated that every cell comes from a cell (i.e. that the cell is the basic unit of life).

Functions of a cell

The cell is a system of cooperative organelles (see below) each carrying out specific functions (Fig. 1.1). In order to survive and reproduce, the cell must maintain an internal environment that sustains biochemical reactions. This homoeostasis is achieved by selectively permeable membranes, separating compartments requiring specific ionic and pH environments.

Cell size is governed by the laws of diffusion, which allow passage of molecules for energy and biosynthesis into the cell and excretion of waste and products across the plasma membrane as follows:

$$\text{Rate of diffusion} \propto (\text{surface area of membrane})^2$$

(If the cell size was too large, the distance the gases would have to diffuse, would be too great to sustain life.)

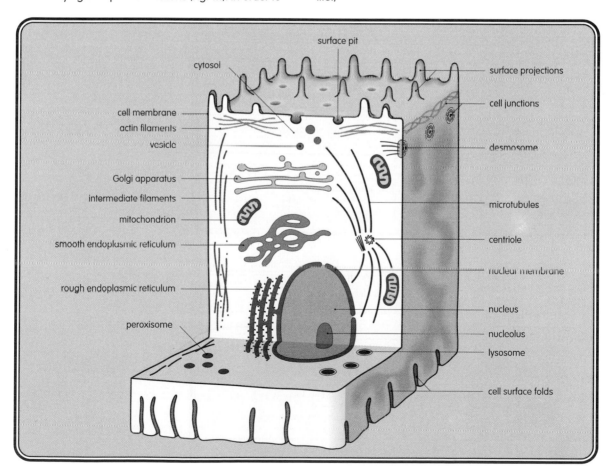

Fig. 1.1 Structure of a typical eukaryotic cell.

Variety of cells

An organism is a system capable of self-replication and self-repair that seeks continually to maintain its complex ordered structure against entropy using a constant flux of energy. Every organism is composed of cells, which are classified into two types—prokaryotic cells and eukaryotic cells (Fig. 1.2).

The genome is located in the nucleus of all somatic cells of multicellular organisms, so all cells are potentially totipotent. Differentiation occurs when individual cells or groups of cells undergo ultrastructural and metabolic changes that distinguish them from other cells in the organism by selective expression of certain genes. In specialization, the structural characteristics of a cell correlate with its function. Examples of specialized cells in humans are shown in Fig. 1.3.

- Define a cell.
- Draw and label a basic cell.
- Define an organism.
- Describe the differences between prokaryotes and eukaryotes—name at least five.

Prokaryotic compared with eukaryotic cells	
Prokaryotic cells	**Eukaryotic cells**
includes bacteria and blue–green algae	four major groups: Protista, fungi, plants and animals
no true nucleus	true nucleus
DNA circular and free	DNA linear and in nucleus
no membrane-bound organelles	internal compartmentalization with organelles, hence division of labour (specialization)
simple binary reproduction	mitotic reproduction (and meiotic)
no development of tissues	tissue and organ systems common
multicellular types rare	independent unicellular organism or part of multicellular organism
size: 1–10 μm	size: 10–100 μm

Fig. 1.2 Prokaryotic compared with eukaryotic cells.

Examples of specialized human cells	
Cell type	**Features**
epithelial cells	shape and size suitable for lining
glandular cells	produce secretions and have a prominent Golgi body
neurons	slender arm-like process transmits electrical impulses
muscle fibres	elongated with abundant contractile proteins that couple electrical activity to contraction
erythrocytes	biconcave discs, no nucleus, loaded with haemoglobin for carrying oxygen

Fig. 1.3 Examples of specialized human cells.

STRUCTURE AND FUNCTION OF CELLULAR ORGANELLES

Concepts

The whole cell is surrounded by the plasma membrane, which forms a dynamic interface between the cytosol and the environment. Cells have a complex ultrastructure comprising membranous and non-membranous organelles. Organelles are structures serving particular functions within the cell.

Membranous organelles

These are enclosed within a phospholipid bilayer and maintain discrete biochemical environments that are optimal for enzymes carrying out specific functions.

Plasma membrane

The plasma membrane is a selectively permeable barrier found on the surface of cells and is responsible for transport between the cell and extracellular fluid by passive diffusion, facilitated diffusion, and active transport (Fig. 1.4). The glycocalyx coat of carbohydrate polymers:

- Produces a negative charge, which separates cells within a multicellular layer.
- Acts as a receptor surface that is sensitive to chemical and other changes in the environment.
- Carries chemical signals enabling other cells (e.g. cells of the immune system) to recognize it.

Microvilli and larger motile cilia project from some cells, for example:

- Microvilli forming the brush border of the small intestine.
- Cilia lining the fallopian tubes and trachea.

Bioelectrical potentials are formed by selective permeability (e.g. nerve cells, muscle cells). Specialized adhesive contacts to other cells include tight junctions, desmosomes, and communicating junctions.

Nucleus

The nucleus:

- Sequesters and replicates DNA.
- Transcribes and splices RNA.
- Allows facilitated selective exchange of molecules up to the size of RNA, e.g. transfer RNA(tRNA), with the cytoplasm.

DNA replication occurs when the genetic code is copied exactly before cell division. In RNA transcription and splicing, genes are decoded and adapted to form a complementary strand of messenger RNA (mRNA), which can be translated into a protein.

Chromosomes are long strands of DNA that carry the genetic code, and chromatin is the combination of DNA with proteins such as histones. Histones inhibit

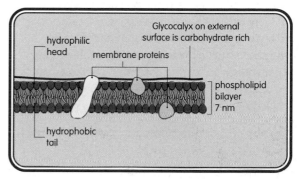

Fig. 1.4 Structure of the plasma membrane.

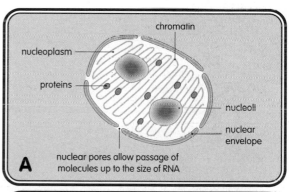

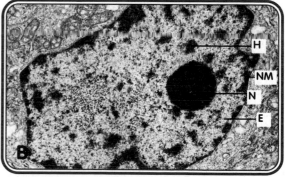

Fig. 1.5 (A) Structure of the nucleus. (B) Electronmicrograph showing the double nuclear membrane (**NM**), nucleolus (**N**), heterochromatin (**H**), which is dense staining, and euchromatin (**E**), which is light staining. (Courtesy of Dr Trevor Gray.)

transcription and replication of DNA, while other DNA-associated proteins function as enzymes for replication, enzymes for transcription, and receptor proteins to detect changes in cytoplasm. Nucleoli are areas within the nucleus where ribosomal RNA is made (Fig. 1.5).

Mitochondria

The structure of a mitochondrion is illustrated in Fig. 1.6. Mitochondria perform aerobic respiration and are self-replicating. Mitochondria originate from primitive bacteria.

Rough (granular) endoplasmic reticulum

Rough endoplasmic reticulum (RER) is a labyrinth of membranous sacs called cisternae, to which enzymes are attached or within which they are contained (Fig. 1.7). Ribosome clusters occur free in the cytoplasm or

attach to the outer surface of the cisternae, where they make polypeptides, which are then in turn:

- Inserted into the membrane.
- Released into the lumen of the cisternae.
- Transported to the Golgi complex or elsewhere.

Proteins made within RER are kept within vesicles or exported to the outside. Cells that make large quantities of secretory protein have large amounts of RER (e.g. pancreatic acinar cells, plasma cells). Free ribosomes synthesize proteins for immediate use in the cytoplasm.

Smooth (agranular) endoplasmic reticulum

Smooth endoplasmic reticulum (SER) is a labyrinth of cisternae, with many enzymes attached to its surface or found within its cisternae. SER:

- Makes steroid hormones (e.g. in the ovary).
- Detoxifies body fluids (e.g. in the liver).

Golgi apparatus

Proteins are modified as they are passed through the Golgi apparatus (e.g. addition of carbohydrate), and are thus 'packaged' for export or storage within the cell. Cells that produce many secretory products have well-developed Golgi apparatus (e.g. hepatocytes). The structure of the Golgi apparatus is shown in Fig. 1.8.

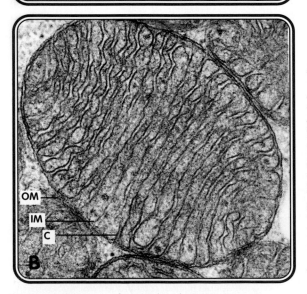

Fig. 1.6 (A) Structure of a mitochondrion. (B) Electronmicrograph showing outer membrane (**OM**), inner membrane (**IM**), and cristae (**C**). (Courtesy of Dr Trevor Gray.)

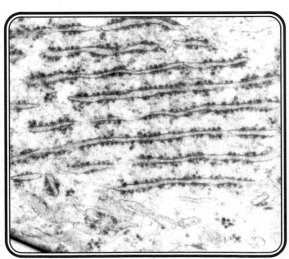

Fig. 1.7 Electronmicrograph of RER. (Courtesy of Dr Trevor Gray.)

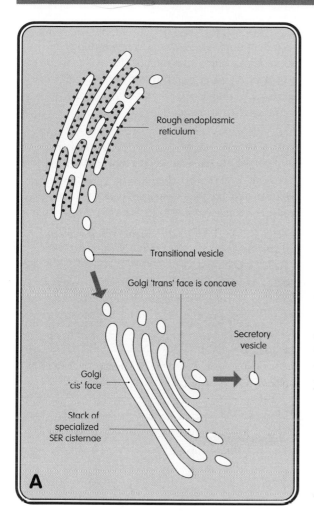

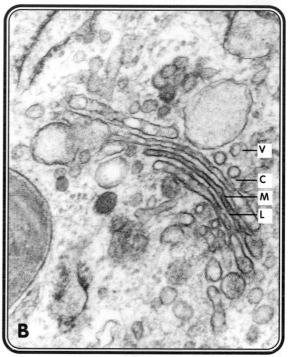

Rough endoplasmic reticulum

Transitional vesicle

Golgi 'trans' face is concave

Secretory vesicle

Golgi 'cis' face

Stack of specialized SER cisternae

A

B

Fig. 1.8 (A) Structure of the Golgi apparatus. (B) Electronmicrograph with parallel stacks of membrane (**M**) delineating Golgi lumen (**L**) from the cytosol (**C**). Transport vesicles (**V**) can be seen on their way from endoplasmic reticulum. (Courtesy of Dr Trevor Gray.)

Fig. 1.9 Electronmicrograph of lysosomes, which are bound by membrane (**M**) and have an electron-dense core composed of acid hydrolase enzymes. (Courtesy of Dr Trevor Gray.)

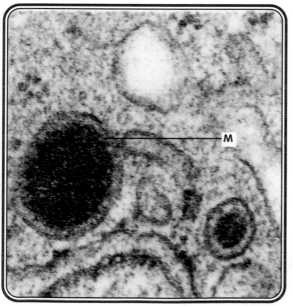

M

Lysosomes

Lysosomes (Fig. 1.9):

- Are vesicular bodies containing granular amorphous material and about 60 types of hydrolytic enzymes.
- Vary in size from 50 nm to over 1 μm.
- Digest material with hydrolases that are active at acid pH.

The multiple pathways of exocytosis, endocytosis, and membrane recycling are illustrated in Fig. 1.10. Autophagy is digestion of material of intracellular origin (e.g. waste products of cell metabolism and redundant organelles), whereas heterophagy is digestion of extracellular material taken into the cell by endocytosis (e.g. bacteria and foreign bodies). Cells specializing in phagocytosis have many lysosomes (e.g. macrophages).

Peroxisomes

Peroxisomes are vesicular bodies that are smaller than lysosomes, and contain enzymes. They perform oxidation and inactivate hydrogen peroxide, which is a product of many metabolic reactions in the cell.

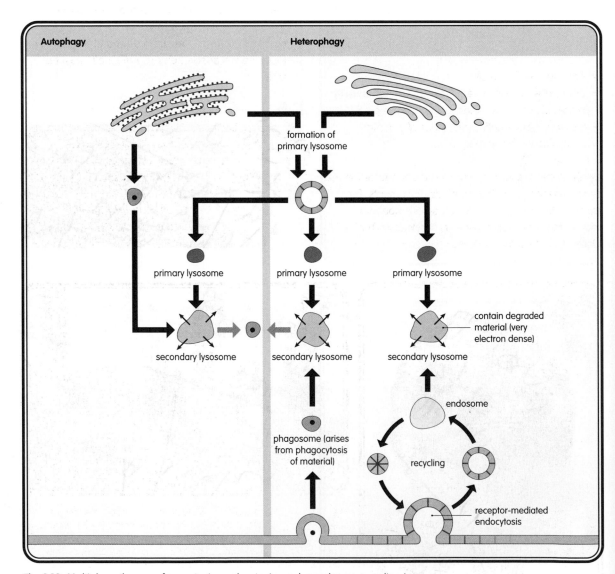

Fig. 1.10 Multiple pathways of exocytosis, endocytosis, and membrane recycling (see also Chapter 4, p. 54.)

Non-membranous organelles
The cytoskeleton

The cytoskeleton is the internal framework of the cell consisting of filaments and tubules. There are several classes of cytoskeletal structures:

- Microfilaments formed from actin.
- Microtubules formed from tubulin.
- Intermediate filaments formed from intermediate filament proteins.

These structures may be crosslinked by other proteins into networks or specialized organelles, the most common of which are:

- Cilia—a '9 + 2' arrangement of microtubules that has a basal body at its base (Fig.1.11). Other filaments are attached, including dynein arms, which bend the cilia via ATP-dependent sliding.
- Flagella—very long cilia.
- Centrioles—which have an identical structure to the basal bodies of cilia and usually occur in pairs.
- Microvilli—non-motile extensions of plasma membrane supported by actin.

Cytoskeletal structures maintain and change cell shape by rearrangement of the cytoskeletal elements, for example by endocytosis, cell division, amoeboid movements, and contraction of muscle cells. Their functions include the following:

The structure and sliding mechanism of cilia are common topics in short-answer questions.

- Ciliary movement is used by some cells to transport substances (e.g. fallopian cells move ova towards the uterus).
- Flagellar movement is used for propulsion (e.g. of spermatozoa).
- Centrioles are responsible for the assembly of microtubules during cell division.
- Microvilli increase the surface area of the cell (e.g. increase the absorption area of small intestine cells)

- Define an organelle.
- Draw and label the histological structures of the major organelles.
- List the functions of individual organelles.

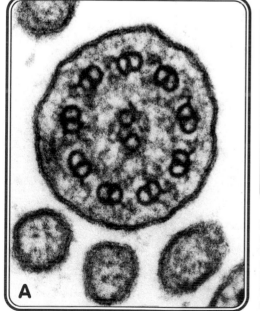

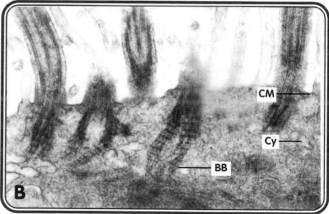

Fig. 1.11 Structure of a cilium (A) Electronmicrograph of traverse-section through a cilium, showing the characteristic 9 + 2 structure of the microtubules. (Courtesy of Dr Trevor Gray.) (B) Electronmicrograph of longitudinal section through the base of a cilium, showing the basal body (**BB**). Here, the outer doublets of the cilium arise directly from the outer triplet of the centriole. (**CM**, cell membrane; **Cy**, cytoplasm) (Courtesy of Dr Trevor Gray.) (See also fig 4.6.)

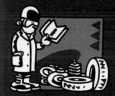

2. Proteins and Enzymes

AMINO ACIDS

Introduction

Amino acids are the subunits of proteins, which all have the same basic structure of:

- A central carbon atom (the α carbon).
- An amino (NH_2) group at the α carbon.
- A carboxyl group (COO).
- A side group (R) (Fig. 2.1).

There are 20 naturally occurring amino acids, which differ in their side group, the simplest being hydrogen (H) in the amino acid glycine. D and L stereoisomer forms exist for all except glycine, as the α carbon is asymmetrical in all but this amino acid (Fig. 2.2). Only the L form is found in humans.

Amino acids form proteins by joining together through peptide bonds to form a polypeptide chain by a process called condensation. There may be a few to several thousand amino acids in a polypeptide, the sequence being determined by the base sequence in DNA. In condensation the amino group of one amino acid and the carboxyl group of another amino group form a peptide bond with the removal of a molecule of water (H_2O) (Fig. 2.3).

The primary structure of a protein is specified by the number and sequence of amino acids in the polypeptide chain. This polypeptide chain may:

- Be further modified by glycosylation or other chemical reactions, which influence its folding.
- Interact with other polypeptides to form a fully biologically active protein.

Essential and non-essential amino acids

There are ten essential and ten non-essential amino acids in human biochemistry:

- Non-essential amino acids are synthesized in the human body, so are not required in the diet.
- Essential amino acids cannot be synthesized by the body, either at all, or at a sufficient rate to meet requirements, so are supplied by dietary protein.

One essential amino acid is required only during growth (arginine), but the others are required throughout life (see *Crash Course Metabolism and Nutrition* for further details.)

Structure of amino acids

The amino acids can be classified by the nature of their R group or side chain (Fig. 2.4).

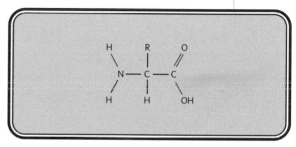

Fig. 2.1 Structure of an amino acid. R is a side group, the simplest being hydrogen (H) in glycine.

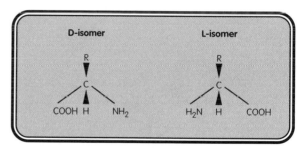

Fig. 2.2 D and L isomers of amino acid.

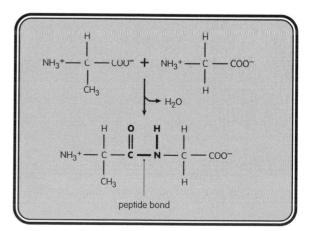

Fig. 2.3 Condensation of amino acids into protein.

Name	Symbol	Stereochemical formula	Side-group type
Aliphatic side chains			
glycine	Gly (G)	$H - CH - COO^-$ $\quad\quad \mid$ $\quad\quad NH_3^+$	small
alanine	Ala (A)	$CH_3 - CH - COO^-$ $\quad\quad\quad \mid$ $\quad\quad\quad NH_3^+$	hydrophobic +
valine	Val (V)	CH_3 $\quad \backslash$ $\quad CH - CH - COO^-$ $\quad /\quad\quad \mid$ $CH_3\quad NH_3^+$	hydrophobic ++
leucine	Leu (L)	CH_3 $\quad \backslash$ $\quad CH - CH_2 - CH - COO^-$ $\quad /\quad\quad\quad\quad \mid$ $CH_3\quad\quad\quad NH_3^+$	hydrophobic +++
isoleucine	Ile (I)	CH_3 $\quad \mid$ $\quad CH_2$ $\quad\quad \backslash$ $\quad\quad CH - CH - COO^-$ $\quad /\quad\quad \mid$ $CH_3\quad NH_3^+$	hydrophobic +++
Aromatic rings			
phenylalanine	Phe (F)	⟨ring⟩$- CH_2 - CH - COO^-$ $\quad\quad\quad\quad\quad \mid$ $\quad\quad\quad\quad\quad NH_3^+$	hydrophobic ++++
tyrosine	Tyr (Y)	$HO -$⟨ring⟩$- CH_2 - CH - COO^-$ $\quad\quad\quad\quad\quad\quad\quad \mid$ $\quad\quad\quad\quad\quad\quad\quad NH_3^+$	hydrophobic (polar)
tryptophan	Trp (W)	⟨indole ring⟩$- CH_2 - CH - COO^-$ $\quad\quad\quad\quad\quad\quad\quad \mid$ $\quad\quad N\quad\quad\quad NH_3^+$ $\quad\quad \mid$ $\quad\quad H$	hydrophobic
Imino acids			
proline	Pro (P)	⟨ring⟩ $\overset{+}{N}$ COO^- $\quad H_2$	closed ring
Acidic groups or amides			
aspartic acid	Asp (D)	$^-OOC - CH_2 - CH - COO^-$ $\quad\quad\quad\quad\quad \mid$ $\quad\quad\quad\quad\quad NH_3^+$	weak acid, pK 4 negative charge

Fig. 2.4 Classification of amino acids by side-group type.

Name	Symbol	Stereochemical formula	Side-group type
Acidic groups or amides (*cont.*)			
asparagine	Asn (N)	$H_2N - C - CH_2 - CH - COO^-$ $\quad\quad \|\| \quad\quad\quad\quad \|$ $\quad\quad O \quad\quad\quad\quad NH_3^+$	polar
glutamic acid	Glu (E)	$^-OOC - CH_2 - CH_2 - CH - COO^-$ $\quad\quad\quad\quad\quad\quad\quad \|$ $\quad\quad\quad\quad\quad\quad\quad NH_3^+$	pK4 negative charge
glutamine	Gln (Q)	$H_2N - C - CH_2 - CH_2 - CH - COO^-$ $\quad\quad \|\| \quad\quad\quad\quad\quad \|$ $\quad\quad O \quad\quad\quad\quad\quad NH_3^+$	polar
Basic groups			
arginine	Arg (R)	$H - N - CH_2 \;\; CH_2 \;\; CH - COO^-$ $\quad\quad \| \quad\quad\quad\quad\quad\quad \|$ $\quad\quad C - NH_2 \quad\quad\quad NH_3^+$ $\quad\quad \|\|$ $\quad\quad NH_2^+$	weak base, pK12 positive charge
lysine	Lys (K)	$CH_2 - CH_2 - CH_2 - CH_2 - CH - COO^-$ $\quad \| \quad\quad\quad\quad\quad\quad\quad\quad \|$ $\quad NH_3^+ \quad\quad\quad\quad\quad\quad NH_3^+$	pK 10 positive charge
histidine	His (H)	$\quad\quad\quad CH_2 - CH - COO^-$ $\quad\quad\quad\quad\quad\quad\quad\quad \|$ $HN \;\; ^+NH \quad\quad\quad NH_3^+$	pK6 positive charge
Hydroxylic groups			
serine	Ser (S)	$CH_2 - CH - COO^-$ $\;\; \| \quad\quad \|$ $\;\; OH \quad NH_3^+$	polar
threonine	Thr (T)	$CH_3 - CH - CH - COO^-$ $\quad\quad\quad \| \quad\quad \|$ $\quad\quad\quad OH \quad NH_3^+$	polar
Sulphur groups			
cysteine	Cys (C)	$\quad\quad\quad H$ $\quad\quad\quad \|$ $NH_3^+ - C - CH_2 - SH$ $\quad\quad\quad \|$ $\quad\quad\quad COO^-$	
methionine	Met (M)	$\quad\quad\quad H$ $\quad\quad\quad \|$ $NH_3^+ - CH_2 - CH_2 - S - CH_3$ $\quad\quad\quad \|$ $\quad\quad\quad COO^-$	

Fig. 2.4 *cont.*

Properties of amino acids

The side chains of amino acids have properties that affect the behaviour of the polypeptide into which they are incorporated.

Size and structure

Larger side chains prevent the chain being bent, and ring structures prevent the chain forming the turns required to make α-helices. Small or hydrophobic amino acids favour the α-helix structure.

Crosslinkages

Links between amino acids occur through hydrogen bonds, disulphide bridges, hydrophobic bonds, and ionic bonds:

- Hydrogen bonds occur between carbonyl (C=O) and imino (N–H) groups.
- Disulphide bridges are covalent bonds between thiol (-SH) groups of cysteine.
- Non-covalent hydrophobic bonds form between two hydrophobic residues.
- Electrovalent (ionic) bonds occur between a negative residue of one amino acid and a positive residue of another amino acid.

Solubility

Hydrophobic side groups cluster in the centre of a protein, while hydrophilic side groups are found on the outside of molecules. Soluble proteins are globular with polar R groups, which attract water (hydrophilic) (e.g. enzymes). Fibrous proteins with non-polar R groups, which repel water (hydrophobic), are insoluble.

Ionization properties of amino acids

Amino acids are amphoteric as they have acidic (negative charge) and basic (positive charge) properties. An amphion is an amino acid in the form where both the acidic and basic properties are expressed with no net charge. At the isoelectric point (pK) for a given amino acid, the pH is such that there is no net charge.

The amino group attracts hydrogen ions, so has basic properties. This is seen in solutions that are more acidic than the pK, where ionization of the carboxyl group is inhibited, giving a net positive electrostatic charge (+1). The acidic property of the amino acid is from the carboxyl group releasing hydrogen ions. In solutions that are more alkaline than the pK, the amino group is inhibited, but the carboxyl group ionizes, giving a net negative electrostatic charge (–1) (Fig. 2.5). If the side chain is an amino group this will attract hydrogen ions in acidic solution, giving an additional positive charge, thus a net charge of +2. If the side chain is an acidic group this will ionize in alkaline solutions, giving an extra negative charge, thus a net charge of –2.

The ability of a protein to accept or donate hydrogen ions is called its buffering capacity. Proteins are important buffers and stabilize the pH of their surroundings, so preventing fluctuations in pH that cannot be tolerated by enzymes in the cell.

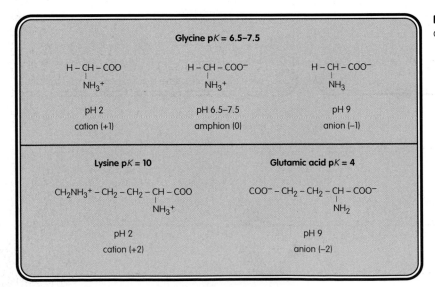

Fig. 2.5 Ionization properties of amino acids.

- Define the basic structure of an amino acid.
- Describe the mechanism of polypeptide formation by condensation.
- Name the classes of amino acids according to their side chains, with examples.
- Discuss the differing properties of the amino acids, with respect to their size and side group.
- Describe the amphoteric nature of amino acids.

PROTEINS

Functions of proteins

Proteins serve a variety of functions in the human body

Functions of proteins	
Protein function	**Examples**
structural	collagen in skin, keratin in hair
metabolism	enzymes (e.g. lysozyme, pepsin, amylase)
signal transduction	cytoplasmic kinases
defence	antibodies
movement	actin and myosin in muscle contraction
transport	haemoglobin carries oxygen, transferrin carries iron
communication	hormones, receptors, and adhesion molecules (e.g. insulin, β-adrenergic receptor, steroid receptor, integrins)
recognition	major histocompatibility complex proteins
storage	ferritin stores iron in the liver

Fig. 2.6 Functions of proteins.

(Fig. 2.6). The shape of the protein is critical to its function, and many proteins have a specific binding site that is of a special shape to fit a ligand, analogous to a lock and key. Examples of such proteins are listed in Fig. 2.7.

Organization of proteins

Primary structure

Primary structure is specified by the linear sequence of amino acids, therefore only peptide bonds are considered. The unique sequence is determined by the bases in DNA. The primary structure (Fig. 2.8) determines the final folded shape.

Proteins and ligands	
Protein	**Ligand**
enzymes	substrate
myosin	actin and other proteins
antibodies	antigen
receptors	hormones, neurotransmitters, counter-receptors

Fig. 2.7 Proteins and ligands.

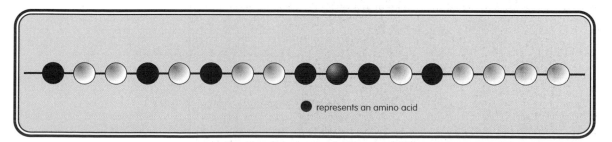

● represents an amino acid

Fig. 2.8 Primary structure of a protein.

15

Secondary structure

Local regions of the polypeptide chain form α helices and β pleated sheets determined by:

- Hydrogen bonding.
- Repulsion of side groups.
- Limited flexibility of the polypeptide chain (Fig. 2.9).

Tertiary structure

Folding occurs to form the unique three-dimensional shape of a polypeptide chain (Fig. 2.10). It is determined by interactions between side groups of the amino acids, including covalent crosslinks (mainly disulphide bridges involving cysteine residues).

Quaternary structure

Two or more polypeptide chains (subunits) associate to form dimers, tetramers, or oligomers (Fig. 2.11). This is required for the protein to show full biological activity.

Forces that shape proteins

Peptide bond

The peptide bond is formed between two amino acids by condensation (see Fig. 2.3). This is a strong covalent bond, which is resistant to heat, pH extremes, and detergent, with a bond energy of 380 kJ/mol^{-1}, and length 0.15 nm or 1.32 Å. The peptide group is planar as it has a partial double-bond character. Consequences of the peptide–bond are as follows:

- The polypeptide chain has restricted flexibility at peptide bonds which are followed by flexible links.
- The partial charge present at the oxygen and nitrogen of the bond enables attraction between two peptide bonds, forming a weak hydrogen bond with a bond energy of 5 kJ/mol.
- Amino acids in a polypeptide are often referred to as 'residues'.

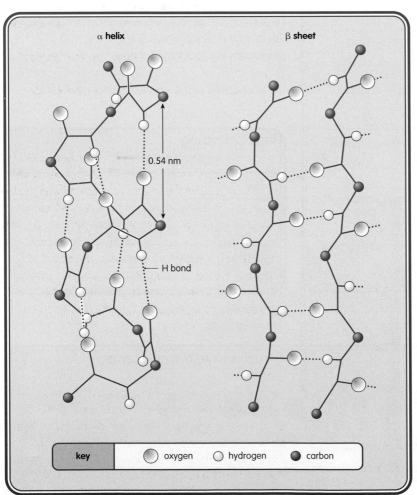

α helix

β sheet

0.54 nm

H bond

| key | | oxygen | | hydrogen | | carbon |

Fig. 2.9 Secondary structure of a protein. In both the α helix and β pleated sheet, regions of secondary structure are stabilized by hydrogen bonds (H bonds) between the C=O and N–H groups of the peptide bonds in the protein.

Hydrogen bonds

Hydrogen bonds occur between peptide bond atoms and polar side groups where a hydrogen atom is shared between two electronegative atoms, and are important in forming coils in secondary structures and the folding of tertiary structures. They have a bond energy of $20\,kJ.mol^{-1}$ and length of $0.3\,nm$ (Fig. 2.12).

Hydrophobic interactions

Hydrophobic residues form interactions rather than true bonds where they cluster close together. Bond energy comes from the displacement of water (e.g. valine, alanine, leucine, and phenylalanine).

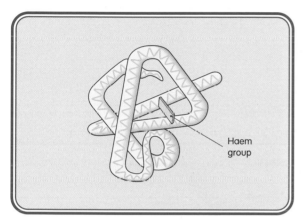

Fig. 2.10 Tertiary structure of a protein. One complete protein chain (β chain of haemoglobin) is illustrated here.

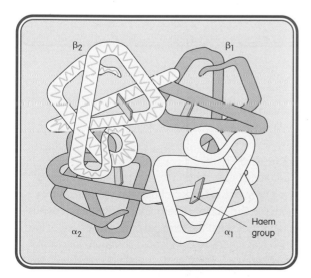

Fig. 2.11 Quaternary structure of a protein. Four separate chains of haemoglobin are assembled into an oligomeric protein.

Ionic interactions

Ionic interactions result from strong attractions between positive and negative atoms. These bonds are seen in tertiary structures and have a bond energy of 335 $kJ.mol^{-1}$ and length of $0.25\,nm$ (see Fig. 2.12).

van der Waals forces

van der Waals forces (dipole-induced dipole) are weak attractions between two atoms as the electron orbitals approach each other (see Fig. 2.12). The bond energy is very weak, being $0.8\,kJ.mol^{-1}$, and the length is $0.35\,nm$. Collectively, these bonds 'add' to significant energy in the tertiary structure of large polypeptides.

Side-chain interactions

Side-chain interactions form bonds, the most important being between the thiol groups of two cysteine residues, forming a covalent bond of $210\,kJ.mol^{-1}$ called a disulphide bridge (see Fig. 2.12). Disulphide bridges are important in tertiary structures and the secondary structure of elastin, and are commonly found in proteins designed for export, for example:

- Digestive enzyme ribonuclease has four disulphide bonds.
- The plasma protein insulin has three disulphide bonds.

Protein folding

The correct 'folded shape' of a protein is determined solely by the amino acid sequence. Chaperone proteins bind to the polypeptide chain and assist in folding to the correct conformation, then detach. Groups far away in the primary sequence may be close together in the final three-dimensional structure. Small conformational changes are possible by mutual rearrangement of helices. A domain is a compact globular unit of the protein made from a specific pattern of α helices and β pleated sheet. Proteins often have defined domains joined by flexible regions.

Structures within proteins
α helix

The α helix discovered by Pauling and Corey in 1951 is a right-handed helix (L form) with a backbone of peptide linkages from which side chains radiate outwards. Small or hydrophobic amino acids favour α helix formation, so glycine or proline are usually found at the α helix bends. The structure is stabilized by hydrogen bonds between every first and fourth amino acid, each hydrogen bond

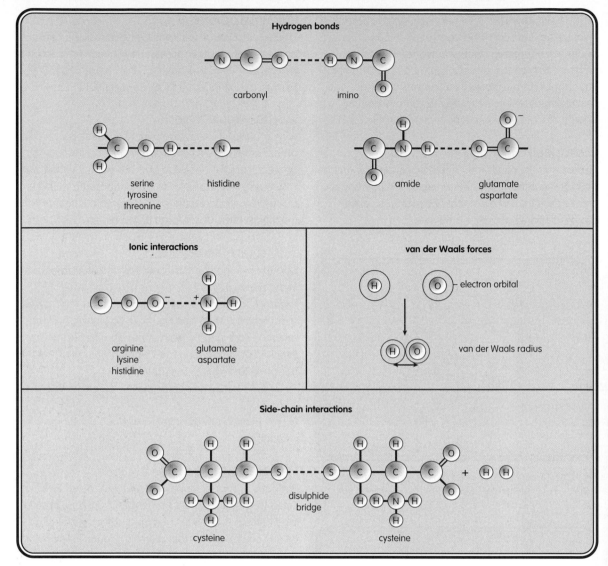

Fig. 2.12 Forces shaping proteins.

being relatively weak, but as all are parallel and 'intrachain' they provide reinforcement. The helix has:

- 0.15 nm rise.
- 0.54 nm pitch.
- 3.6 residues per turn.

The structure is a rigid rod-like cylinder that is very stable, with side groups pointing out and therefore free to interact with other α helices (see Fig. 2.9). α helices make up 90–100% of fibrous proteins and 10–60% of globular proteins, for example:

- α-keratin, a fibrous protein in hair of α helices fur, and wool, formed from side-to-side packing of α

helices into a superhelix.
- Myoglobin, a globular protein.

β pleated sheet

β pleated sheets, which were discovered by Pauling and Corey, are extended chains formed from two or more pleated polypeptides joined by hydrogen bonds. In a parallel sheet the terminal amino acids are at the same end whereas, in the more common antiparallel sheet, terminal amino acids are at opposite ends, so forming a more stable structure (see Fig. 2.9). The sheet is a rigid non-elastic 'platform', which is commonly found in fibrous proteins, for example:

- β–keratins in claws, scales, feathers, and beaks are made of antiparallel strands.
- Silk is made of regular β sheets.

Bonds between the sheets give tensile strength, but flexibility due to slipping of one layer over the layer below.

Elastin
Elastin is a connective tissue with great elasticity and is formed from three to seven α helices wound around each other and connected by disulphide bridges. Unstretched it exists as random coils, but once stretched it forms a regular shape.

Collagen
The collagen helix has great strength, but little elasticity; its three polypeptide chains are interconnected by hydrogen bonds and permanently extended.

Zinc fingers
Zinc fingers, a common motif in many DNA-binding proteins, have special 'zinc finger domains', which are folded amino acid projections surrounding a central zinc atom. They recognize specific DNA sequences (Fig. 2.13).

Stability of proteins
Denaturation is loss of the three-dimensional structure of a protein due to breaking of some of the structural bonds (Fig. 2.14). Most proteins function only within narrow environmental limits, with denaturing conditions being beyond these limits (e.g. heat, pH extremes, detergents, oxidation, and physical effects such as shaking). If the conditions are not extreme, the protein may return to its active state when returned to optimal conditions.

Complex structures
Many proteins have additional molecules added after synthesis, which may themselves be proteins or other molecules.
- A prosthetic group is an essential organic group or other atom that is conjugated to a protein molecule, for example:
- Iron-containing haem in haemoglobin.
- Vitamin A with the photoreceptor rhodopsin.
- Other cofactor non-protein components required for a protein to function may be unattached as free metal ions or coenzyme.
- Coenzymes are non-protein, but are organic (made of carbon and hydrogen). Carbohydrate or lipid may also be added, for example:
- Glycoproteins in the plasma membrane assist adhesion.
- Lipoproteins enable lipid transport in the plasma.

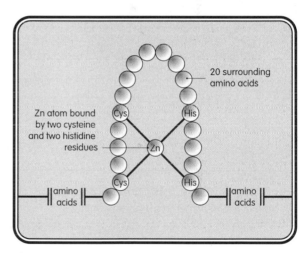

Fig. 2.13 Zinc finger domain.

Fig. 2.14 Denaturation of protein.

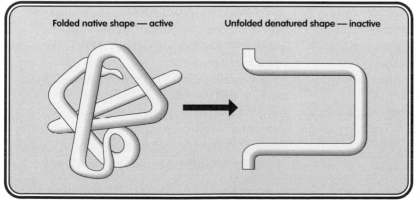

19

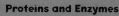

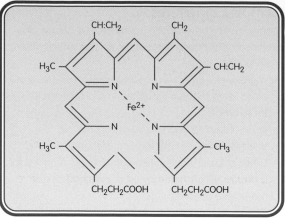

Fig. 2.15 Structure of haem.

- **Describe the main functions of proteins, with examples—be able to list at least five.**
- **Define what is meant by primary, secondary, tertiary, and quaternary protein structure.**
- **Discuss the six major bonds found in proteins (peptide bonds, hydrogen bonds, hydrophobic bonds, ionic interactions, van der Waals forces, and side-chain with respect to their properties, bond energy, and consequences, and name examples.**
- **Describe the structural properties of α helices, β pleated sheets, elastin, collagen helix, and zinc fingers.**
- **Define prosthetic group, cofactor, and coenzyme.**

Protein structure and folding are commonly asked about in essay questions.

Interactions between subunits are important to the function of the multimer (e.g. haemoglobin A in normal adults is composed of two α subunits and two β subunits, each associated with a prosthetic haem group (Fig. 2.15).

Haem is a porphyrin that combines with oxygen. When oxygen joins the first haem group it causes a change in the bonding affinity of the second haem group via conformational changes in the globin chains. This enables the second haem to combine rapidly with an oxygen molecule, which in turn alters the third haem. Thus the polypeptide chains control the oxygen-carrying capacity of haem.

Protein isoforms are proteins with identical biological activity, but different structures or amino acid sequences, for example:
- Myosin in heart tissue.
- Myosin in fast muscle fibres.

ENZYMES

Introduction
In 1876 Kuhne coined the word enzyme, which literally means 'in yeast', as juice from yeast was shown to cause fermentation. Enzymes are simple or conjugated proteins that act as biological catalysts, increasing the rate of a reaction without themselves undergoing chemical change. Intracellular enzymes control cell metabolism; extracellular enzymes are made inside the cell, but act outside it.

An enzyme's name is normally the name of the substrate with the suffix -ase added, the substrate being the substance on which the enzyme acts. Isoenzymes catalyse the same reaction, but have different structures, for example:
- Lactate dehydrogenase has heart and muscle isoforms.
- Creatine kinase has brain and muscle isoforms.

Classification of enzymes

There are six main classes of enzymes.

Oxidoreductases

Oxidoreductases oxidize substrates, and are either oxidases or dehydrogenases.

Dehydrogenases

Dehydrogenases transfer hydrogen to coenzymes:

substrate + coenzyme $\rightarrow$ oxidized substrate + reduced coenzyme

$AH_2 + 2NAD^+ \rightarrow A^+ + 2NADH$

For example, alcohol dehydrogenase catalyzes:

$$\text{ethanol} \rightarrow \text{acetaldehyde}$$
$$CH_3CH_2OH + NAD^+ \rightarrow CH_3\text{-}C{=}O + NADH + H^+$$
$$\phantom{CH_3CH_2OH + NAD^+ \rightarrow CH_3\text{-}C{=}O}\overset{|}{H}$$

Oxidases

Oxidases transfer hydrogen to oxygen molecules:

substrate $\rightarrow$ oxidized substrate

$AH_2 + 1/2\ O_2 \rightarrow A + H_2O$

For example, cytochrome oxidase catalyses:

Cyt.H_2 (reduced cytochrome) $+ 1/2\ O_2 \rightarrow$
Cyt$+ H_2O$ (cytochrome)

Transferases

Transferases move molecules from one substrate to another, for example kinases transfer phosphate groups:

$AB + C \rightarrow A + BC$

For example, glucokinase catalyses:

D-Glucose + ATP $\rightarrow$ D-Glucose-6-phosphate + ADP

Hydrolases

Hydrolases form two products from a single substrate by hydrolysis, coupling the hydrogen atom from water to one component and the hydroxyl group to another:

$AB + H_2O \rightarrow AH + BOH$

For example, carboxypeptidase A catalyzes:

$$\begin{array}{c} R_{n-1}\quad O\quad\ R_n \\ -N-C-C-N-C-COO^- + H_2O \\ \ \ H\ \ H\quad\ \ H\ \ H \end{array}$$

C-terminal of polypeptide

$$\downarrow$$

$$\begin{array}{cc} R_{n-1} & R_n \\ -N-C-COO^- \qquad + \qquad H_3{}^+N-C-COO^- \\ \ \ H\ \ H & \qquad\qquad\ \ H \end{array}$$

polypeptide shortened   *C*-terminal residue

Lyases

Lyases break down C–C bonds. Two simpler products are formed as with hydrolases, but water is not involved:

$AB \rightarrow A + B$

For example pyruvate decarboxylase catalyzes:

$$\overset{O}{\overset{\|}{^-OOC\text{-}C\text{-}CH_3}} + H^+ \rightarrow CO_2 + \overset{O}{\overset{\|}{C\text{-}CH_3}}$$
$$\qquad\qquad\qquad\qquad\qquad\qquad\ \overset{|}{H}$$

pyruvate   acetaldehyde

Isomerases

Isomerases change the isomeric configuration of a molecule, so transfer atoms from one part of the molecule to another:

$ABC \rightarrow ACB$

For example, maleate isomerase catalyzes:

$$\begin{array}{cc} ^-OOC\quad COO^- & ^-OOC\quad\ H \\ \diagdown\ \ / & \diagdown\ \ / \\ C{=}C \quad\rightarrow & C{=}C \\ /\quad\ \ \diagdown & /\qquad \diagdown \\ H\qquad\ H & H\qquad COO^- \end{array}$$

malate   fumarate

Ligases

Ligases form new bonds, with energy provided by ATP:

$A + B + ATP \rightarrow AB + ADP + P$

For example pyruvate carboxylase catalyzes:

$$\overset{O}{\overset{\|}{^-OOC\text{-}C\text{-}CH_3}} + CO_2 + ATP \rightarrow \overset{O}{\overset{\|}{^-OOC\text{-}C\text{-}CH_2\text{-}COO^-}} + ADP + P$$

pyruvate   oxaloacetate

Properties of enzymes

Enzymes have a high catalytic efficiency

Enzymes increase the rate of reactions without being consumed, and, without enzymes, metabolic reactions would be too slow for life. The turnover rate is the number of substrate molecules that one enzyme molecule turns into product per minute. Catalase is the fastest enzyme, with a turnover rate of six million operations per minute; most enzymes, have a rate of several thousand. Enzymes are more efficient than inorganic catalysts, owing to their lower activation energy (Fig. 2.16).

Enzymes are reusable

Enzymes are not consumed by the reactions they catalyse: they can be used again; however, unlike inorganic catalysts they are not stable, so cannot be used indefinitely and must be constantly replaced.

Enzymes work in both directions

The direction a chemical reaction proceeds in depends upon the amounts of the substrate and products present:

$$K_{eq} = \frac{[C]}{[A][B]}$$

Enzymes speed up the reaction in either direction until equilibrium is achieved. The equilibrium point and energy change of the reaction (ΔG) are not altered.

Enzymes are highly specific

Enzymes usually catalyse only one type of reaction, acting on one particular optical isomer or isolated chemical group. Intracellular enzymes normally have only one substrate, while extracellular enzymes usually act on a group of related substrates.

Some enzymes contain non-protein cofactors

Cofactors are sometimes required for enzyme activity and are commonly metal ions (e.g. Zn^{2+}, Fe^{2+}) or vitamin derivatives (e.g. nicotinamide adenine dinucleolide [NAD], flavine adenine dinucleolide [FAD]).

Enzyme activity is regulated

Many reactions take place in an individual cell, and need to be organized. Specificity of enyzmes constitutes one method of regulation; others are activation or inhibition by allosteric modifiers or covalent modification of the enzyme itself.

Lock-and-key hypothesis

This hypothesis was proposed by Fuscher in 1894, to explain how enzymes act. It states that the enzyme and substrate combine to form an enzyme–substrate complex, with the substrate molecules held in such a way that new bonds are formed (enzyme–product complex); finally, the enzyme dissociates from the product and can be used again:

The active site is the place on the enzyme where

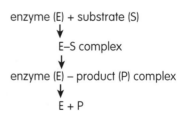

enzyme (E) + substrate (S)
↓
E–S complex
↓
enzyme (E) – product (P) complex
↓
E + P

Fig. 2.16 Decreased activation energy with catalyzed reaction. AB are the substrates, C is the product.

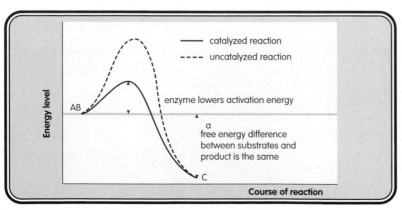

— catalyzed reaction
---- uncatalyzed reaction

Energy level

AB

enzyme lowers activation energy

a
free energy difference between substrates and product is the same

C

Course of reaction

substrate binds; its shape and chemical groups mean that only substrate with a complementary structure can combine, analogous to a lock and key. The lock-and-key hypothesis explains why enzymes are specific and how activation energy is lowered. When the substrate binds to the enzyme, its bond angles are distorted, so less energy is required to break them. Koshland proposed the 'induced fit' hypothesis in 1968 to explain the action of some enzymes where substrate binding to the enzyme changes the conformation of the active site (Fig. 2.17).

Structure of enzymes

Over 90% of enzymes are globular proteins and the rest are conjugated to a prosthetic group. Recent studies by X-ray diffraction and other techniques have advanced knowledge about the structure of enzymes and provided evidence for the lock-and-key and induced-fit hypotheses. The structure of lactate dehydrogenase is known in detail—it has:

• Two globular domains.

• One nucleotide-binding domain.
• A second catalytic domain (Fig. 2.18).

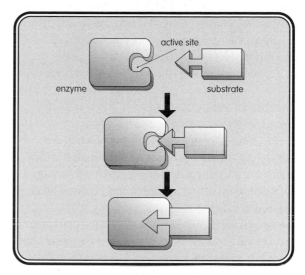

Fig. 2.17 The 'induced fit' hypothesis explains how the binding of the substrate to the enzyme changes the conformation of the active site.

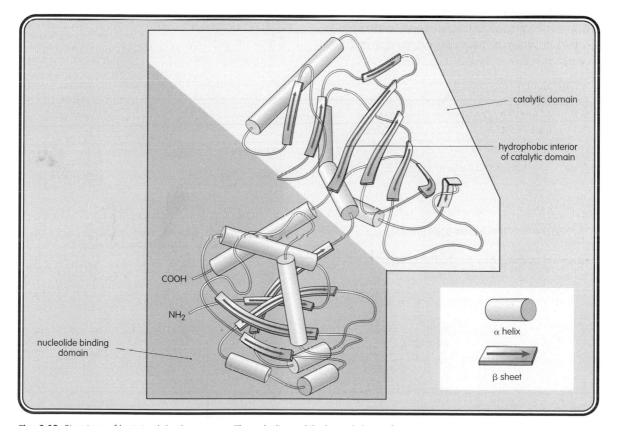

Fig. 2.18 Structure of lactate dehydrogenase. The α helix and β pleated sheets form two globular binding domains.

The nucleotide (cofactor) binding domain has a β–α–β turn that promotes NAD binding, which is conserved in all known NAD- or NADPH-dependent dehydrogenases (Fig. 2.19). This domain also has:

- Positive charges on arginine side chains, which attract the negative phosphate groups of cofactors.
- Glycines for turn tightness, NAD binding, and interactions between the α helix and β strands.

The domain undergoes induced fit. The β–α–β loop moves 1.4 nm upon NAD or NADP binding.

The catalytic domain has a hydrophobic pocket, which has a specific three-dimensional shape for the substrate, and charged residues, which are important for substrate binding. Conformational changes bring the bound substrate into close proximity to the nicotinamide ring. The conformation of the active site favours the transition state. Amino acid side chains and cofactors participate in catalysis, but electron transfer catalyses the reaction (Fig. 2.20).

Enzyme kinetics

Enzyme kinetics is the study of the rate of change of reactants and products. Enzyme assays use biosensors, oxygen electrodes, chromogenic substances, and other methods to measure the progress of reactions.

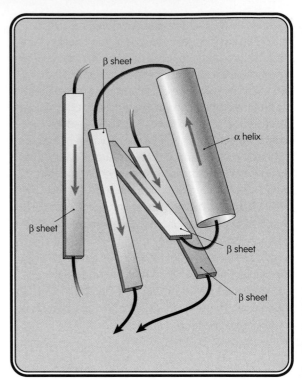

Fig. 2.19 Core structure of the nucleotide cofactor binding domain. All NAD-or NAPH-dependent dehydrogenases have a similar binding domain.

Fig. 2.20 Hydrophobic pocket of catalytic domain.

Reaction rates

By plotting the amount of product formed against time, the initial velocity of the reaction can be estimated (Fig. 2.21A). The initial velocity (V) equals the reaction rate. Reaction rate varies according to enzyme and substrate concentration. Increasing enzyme concentration increases the reaction linearly, so follows first order kinetics (Fig. 2.21B).

Increasing substrate concentration increases the reaction rate in an asymptotic, non linear, fashion; as the enzyme becomes saturated the reaction rate reaches a limit—this is a Michaelis–Menten graph (Fig. 2.22). For simple enzymes the curve is a rectangular hyperbola. At low substrate concentrations the graph is linear (rate is proportional to [substrate]), so follows first order kinetics. At high substrate concentrations a plateau is reached, so follows zero order kinetics. The Michaelis–Menten equation relates the enzyme rate to the substrate concentration:

$$E + S \underset{K_2}{\overset{K_1}{\rightleftharpoons}} ES \underset{K_4}{\overset{K_3}{\rightleftharpoons}} E + P$$

K_4 is insignificant so is ignored.

The Michaelis constant (K_m) is the rate of breakdown of the enzyme–substrate complex:

$$K_m = \frac{(K_2 + K_3)}{K_1}$$

The maximum velocity (V_{max}) is reached under saturating conditions when the substrate concentration is high:

$$V_{max} = K_3[ES]$$

where K_3 is rate of enzyme and product formation and [ES] is enzyme–product complex concentration.

The velocity (V) of a Michaelis–Menten reaction is therefore:

$$V = \frac{V_{max} \times [S]}{K_m + [S]}$$

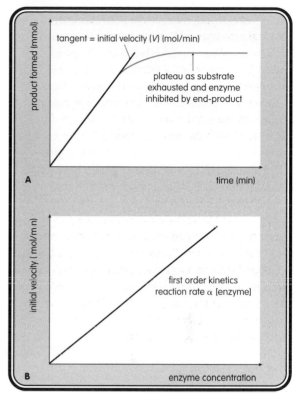

Fig. 2.21 (A) Calculation of initial velocity. (B) Effect of enzyme concentration on reaction rate. (V, initial velocity.)

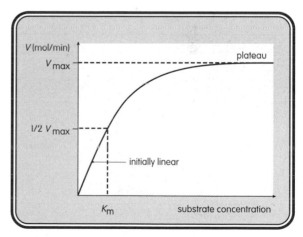

Fig. 2.22 Michaelis–Menten graph showing effect of increasing substrate concentration against reaction rate. (K_m, Michaelis constant; V_{max}, maximum velocity.)

- V_{max} and K_m are constants for each different enzyme.
- For most enzymes, K_m is the substrate concentration at which the reaction rate is half of V_{max}.
- K_m is a measure of the affinity of the enzyme for its substrate, with a low K_m (low enzyme–substrate complex breakdown) corresponding to high affinity (tight binding) and vice versa.
- V_{max} and K_m are difficult to estimate from a Michaelis–Menten graph, so an alternative graph representation is used, the Lineweaver–Burk graph (Fig. 2.23).

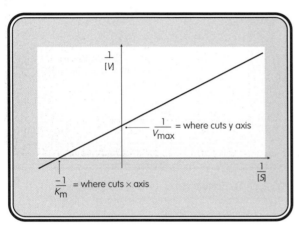

Fig. 2.23 Lineweaver–Burk plot. (K_m, Michaelis constant, S, substrate; V, velocity; V_{max}, maximum velocity.)

Inhibitors

Enzyme inhibitors are substances that lower enzyme activity. False inhibitors include denaturing treatments and irreversible inhibitors (e.g. organophosphorus compounds). True inhibitors are either:

- Competitive.
- Non-competitive.
- Allosteric.

Competitive inhibitors resemble the substrate, and compete for the active site (Fig. 2.24A). The K_m is increased, so affinity of the enzyme is decreased; for example azidothymidine (AZT) used to treat HIV resembles deoxythymidine, so is a competitive inhibitor of the HIV virus reverse transcriptase.

Non-competitive inhibitors (e.g. heavy metals such as lead) do not resemble the substrate, so do not compete for the binding site. They bind to the enzyme and abolish its catalytic activity, although substrate may still bind (Fig. 2.24B). V_{max} is decreased, as there is less catalytically active enzyme, but K_m is unchanged as affinity of the enzyme is not altered.

Allosteric inhibitors do not bind to the active site; instead they bind to a different allosteric site elsewhere on the enzyme. Binding causes a conformational change, which can alter V_{max} and/or K_m; for example phosphofructokinase I (PFK I) is allosterically inhibited by high concentrations of ATP and by citrate (Fig. 2.25).

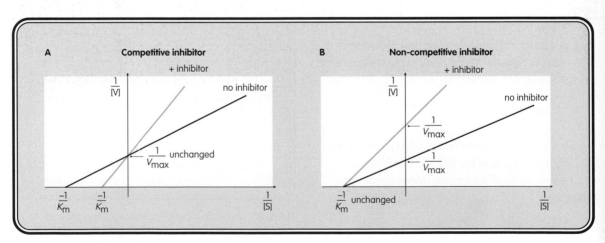

Fig. 2.24 (A) Competitive inhibition of enzyme. The inhibitor increases K_m, and V_{max} is unchanged. (B) Non-competitive inhibition of enzyme. The inhibitor decreases V_{max} and K_m remains unchanged. (K_m, Michaelis constant, S, substrate; v, velocity; V_{max}, maximum velocity)

Clinical significance of genetic variation of enzyme function

Genetic variation of enzyme function can have clinical consequences:

- The cholinesterase enzyme may be functionally altered if there is a mutation in its gene located on chromosome 3. This enzyme normally metabolizes suxamethonium, a short-acting induction agent used in anaesthesia. A mutant form fails to act on the drug, resulting in prolonged paralysis and apnoea.
- The glucose-6-phosphate dehydrogenase enzyme is encoded on the X chromosome and protects erythrocytes from oxidative damage. Variations in this enzyme can cause a haemolytic anaemia

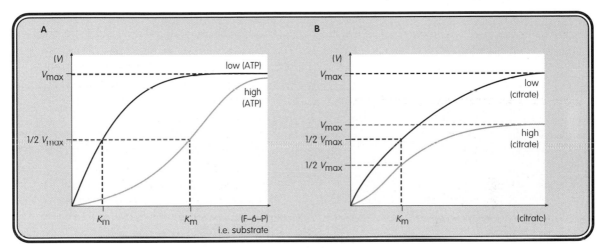

Fig. 2.25 Allosteric inhibition of PFK 1 (A) ATP increases K_m (decreases affinity), but does not alter V_{max}. (B) Citrate decreases V_{max}, but does not alter K_m. (K_m, Michaelis constant; S, substrate; V, velocity; V_{max}, maximum velocity.)

- Define an enzyme, catalyst, substrate, and isoenzyme.
- Name the seven classes of enzymes, with examples.
- Discuss the 'lock and key' and 'induced fit' hypotheses.
- Describe a typical Michaelis–Menten graph and Lineweaver–Burk graph.
- What are the effects of each class of inhibitor on enzyme kinetics?

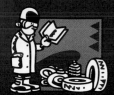

3. The Cell Membrane

Fluid mosaic model

The fluid mosaic model of biological membranes was proposed by Singer and Nicholson in 1972. The membrane is 6–10 nm wide. Verification of the fluid mosaic model has been shown by freeze fracture and freeze etching electron microscope techniques, which show the distribution of proteins within the membrane. The lipids form a bilayer with a consistency similar to that of machine oil. The lipid is stabilized by:

- Hydrophobic interactions of the bilayer interior.
- Hydrophilic interactions of polar head groups with the aqueous environment.

Phospholipids are the major lipid component of the plasma membrane (Fig. 3.1).

The proteins are classified as peripheral or integral. Peripheral proteins are stabilized by electrostatic interactions with the lipid surface, and are easily extracted. Integral proteins undergo hydrophobic interactions with the lipid, so are difficult to extract without disrupting the membrane.

A lipid is a molecule of biological origin that is soluble in an organic solvent (e.g. chloroform), but only sparingly soluble in water. Triglycerides contain a glycerol esterified to fatty acids, and are not found in

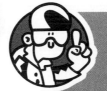

The fluid mosaic model is a common topic in exams; remember to draw a diagram, even for short-answer questions. Remember that the membrane is not fixed. Imagine the cell membrane structure as a sea of lipids, with protein 'icebergs' floating within it and able to diffuse through it.

the lipid membrane. Fatty acids are carboxylic acid with variable length hydrocarbon side chains.

Components of the biological membrane

Phospholipids

Phospholipids contain one glycerol molecule, one phosphate group, and two fatty acid groups (Fig. 3.2). There are four major phospholipids in the plasma membrane:

- Phosphatidylethanolamine.
- Phosphatidylserine.
- Phosphatidylcholine.
- Sphingomyelin.

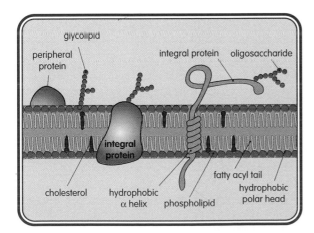

Fig. 3.1 Fluid mosaic model of the cell membrane.

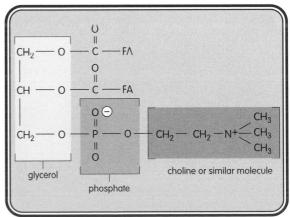

Fig. 3.2 Structure of a phospholipid. (FA, fatty acid.)

The first two occur in the outer portion of the membrane, and the second two in the inner portion of the membrane (Fig. 3.3). Sphingomyelin is not a true phospholipid, but a sphingolipid with a choline group attached via a phosphate molecule to a ceramide (which consists of sphingosine plus a fatty acid tail).

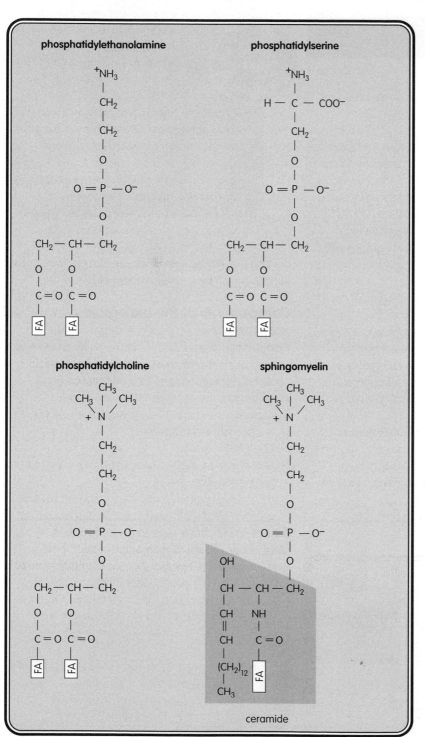

Fig. 3.3 The four major phospholipids. (FA, fatty acid.)

The phospholipids were shown by Sir Hardy in 1918 to be amphipathic—that is, they have hydrophobic and hydrophilic regions. Most lipids pack as cylinders or slightly truncated cones. Fatty acids influence the packing; thus lysophospholipids, which have one fatty acid missing, are shaped like cones and form micelles if there is membrane lysis (Fig. 3.4).

Cholesterol

Cholesterol is a lipid and is the most abundant steroid

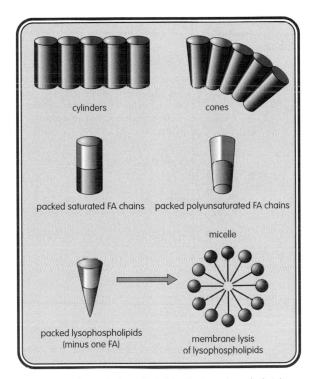

cylinders   cones

packed saturated FA chains   packed polyunsaturated FA chains

micelle

packed lysophospholipids (minus one FA)   membrane lysis of lysophospholipids

Fig. 3.4 Packing of phospholipids. On lysophospholipid membrane lysis micelles are produced. (FA, fatty acid.)

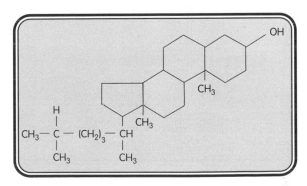

Fig. 3.5 Structure of cholesterol.

in the membrane and influences the fluidity of the membrane (Fig. 3.5).

Membrane proteins

There are three main types of membrane proteins:

- Integral proteins, which span the membrane with contact outside and inside the cell.
- Anchored (peripheral) proteins, which are loosely associated with the membrane and have only one orientation.
- Surface-associated membrane proteins, which are always on the outside of the membrane, giving charge and functioning as receptors.

Integral proteins may pass through the membrane many times. Monotopic proteins pass through the membrane once, while bitopic and polytopic proteins have polypeptide chains which pass through the membrane twice and many times, respectively. Integral proteins traverse the membrane as α helical loops, and hairpin when they cross repeatedly (Fig. 3.25).

Peripheral membrane proteins are attached to the plasma membrane by attachment to another protein or covalent modification of lipids at either:

- The inner face (e.g. *ras* a messenger G protein that transfers signals from the membrane to molecules in the cytoplasm is bound by a thioester bond to farnesyl).
- The extracellular face (e.g. glycoprotein I anchors a number of proteins).

Examples of membrane proteins and their functions are listed in Fig. 3.6.

Peripheral membrane proteins can be dissociated from the membrane by relatively mild procedures that leave the membrane intact (e.g. cytochrome *c*). Dissociation of integral membrane proteins poses a problem as the cell membrane and membrane proteins are both very hydrophobic. Separation can only be achieved by agents that disrupt the membrane, so detergents are used to solubilize and remove the proteins. Specific detergents vary in their solubilizing and denaturing effects:

- Non-ionic detergents (e.g. octylglucoside) are gentle, but not very solubilizing.
- Ionic detergents (e.g. sodium deoxycholate) are good at solubilizing, but are quite denaturing, so may unfold the protein.

Membrane proteins and their functions		
Integral protein	**Function**	**Importance**
LDL receptor	binds LDL	abnormal in familial hypercholesterolaemia
gap junction connexin subunit	transport	transport of small molecules between cells
peripheral gangliosides	receptors	toxin can bind the receptor, so it is taken into the cell where it has effects (e.g. grossly disturbed ion balance when cholera toxin binds to its receptor Gm1 in the intestine)
oncogene	signal transduction	important in the mechanism of neoplasia (e.g. *ras*)

Fig. 3.6 Examples of membrane proteins and their functions. (LDL, low-density lipotrotein.)

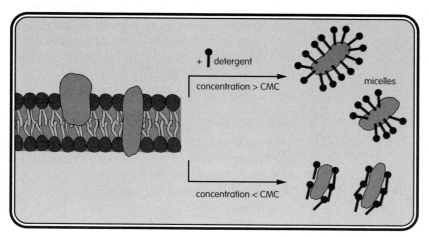

Fig. 3.7 Effect of detergent concentration and critical micelle concentration (CMC) on micelle formation.

Increasing detergent concentration increases the probability that the hydrophobic region of the protein will be bound. Detergents have a given critical micelle concentration (CMC), which is the concentration required to solubilize membrane proteins as micelles (Fig. 3.7). A micelle is a globular aggregation of hydrocarbon groups out of contact with water, so permits solvation of polar groups. A detergent with a high CMC may dissociate membrane proteins without forming micelles as it will dissolve the membrane at a concentration below its CMC.

Properties of biological membranes
Fluidity
Phospholipids determine the fluidity of the membrane and are influenced by temperature, saturation of fatty acid chains and cholesterol.

As the lipid bilayer cools below its transition temperature it becomes a gel-like solid (Fig. 3.8). Body temperature is above the transition temperature, so the membrane is fluid.

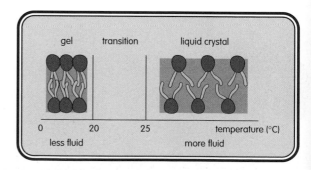

Fig. 3.8 Membrane transition from gel to liquid crystal.

The transition temperature increases with chain length and degree of saturation. As the degree of polyunsaturation increases, the fluidity increases (Fig. 3.9). Saturated fatty acids have a higher melting point due to hydrogen bonds forming dimers, thus fluidity decreases. The distribution of lipids in the membrane is uneven, with ordered regions alternating with more fluid regions.

Cholesterol decreases membrane fluidity at body temperature as it interferes with mobility of the fatty acid side chains. Increasing cholesterol concentration causes increased membrane rigidity as it has a fused ring structure; this hardening is important in atherosclerosis. Fluidity allows membrane proteins to interact.

Mobility of membrane components

Phospholipid molecules rarely undergo transverse diffusion through the lipid bilayer. The asymmetrical orientation of integral proteins is maintained by their flip-flop rates of between four hours and 30 days as a result of their 'head groups' being larger than those of lipids; specialized membrane proteins catalyse flip-flops (flipases). Lipid molecules are, however, highly mobile in the plane of the bilayer and lateral diffusion is freely possible at a rate of 10^{-8} cm^2/s.

Proteins are also mobile and this can be shown by fluorescence photo bleaching in which the cell is bleached so fluorescent antibodies to cell proteins can be seen to move. In some cases membrane components are not free to diffuse in the plane of the membrane (e.g. acetylcholine receptors at the motor end plate). Restriction of mobility of the proteins is by anchorage to cytoskeletal components (e.g. spectrin). Cholesterol diminishes the lateral mobility of lipids and proteins in the membrane.

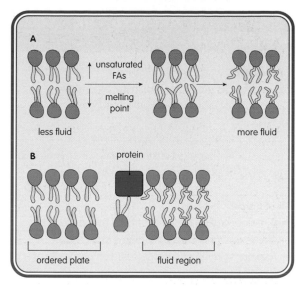

Fig. 3.9 Factors affecting membrane fluidity. (A) Increasing the concentration of unsaturated fatty acids (FAs) decreases the melting point of the membrane and so increases fluidity. (B) Uneven distribution of membrane lipids affects the fluidity.

Permeability

There are three main forms of transport across the membrane:

- Passive diffusion.
- Facilitated diffusion.
- Active transport.

Lipid bilayers are permeable to lipid-soluble compounds, but very impermeable to ionic and polar substances, which require dedicated channels to cross the membrane. Although polar, water is membrane permeable because it is a very small molecule.

○ **Draw a labelled diagram of the fluid mosaic model.**
○ **Discuss the two major classes of membrane proteins and their dissociation.**
○ **What are the properties of the plasma membrane (list three)?**
○ **Discuss the effect of cholesterol on the membrane, and its clinical significance.**

TRANSPORT ACROSS THE CELL MEMBRANE

Concepts

Concentrations are measured in moles and the dissociation of ions is not taken into account.

$$1 \text{ mole} = 6.02 \times 10^{23} \text{ molecules (of any kind)}$$
$$= \text{Avogadro's constant (the number of atoms in exactly 12g of carbon 12)}$$

For example:
- A molar solution of NaCl contains one mole of Na atoms and one mole of Cl atoms in 1L.
- A molar solution of sucrose contains one mole of sucrose in 1L.
- A molar solution of $CaCl_2$ contains one mole of Ca^{2+} and two moles of Cl in 1L.

Osmosis is the movement of molecules across a semipermeable membrane from a region of high concentration to a region of low concentration. The osmotic pressure is the pressure required to prevent the net movement of pure water into an aqueous solution through a semipermeable membrane. In osmotic pressure the dissociation of ions is important.

$$1 \text{ osmole} = 10^{23} \text{ osmotically active particles}$$

For example:
- One osmol/L of NaCl contains 0.5 moles of the ion Na^+ and 0.5 moles of the ion of Cl^-.
- One osmol/L of sucrose contains one mole of sucrose.
- Three osmol/L of $CaCl_2$ contains one mole of the ion Ca^{2+} and two moles of the ion Cl^-.

The osmolarity of plasma is critical, as changes affect plasma volume, cell volume, and water and ion homoeostasis:
- Isotonic extracellular solutions have the same osmotic pressure as the inside of the cell, so osmosis does not occur.
- Hypotonic solutions are less concentrated, so water will pass into the cell.
- Hypertonic solutions are more concentrated, so water will pass out of the cell.

Normal plasma osmolarity is approximately 0.3 osmol/L (i.e. 300 mosmol/L). K^+, Na^+, and Cl^- are fully dissociated, whereas Ca^{2+}, Mg^{2+}, and H^+ are only partially dissociated in living systems. Dissociation is affected by pH, temperature, and binding of ions to compounds (e.g. Ca^{2+} binding to myosin during muscle contraction).

Distribution of ions across the cell membrane

The distribution of various ions across the cell membrane is shown in Fig. 3.10. It is maintained by:
- The semipermeable membrane concept.
- The Gibbs–Donnan equilibrium.
- Pores, channels, and pumps.

Semipermeable membrane concept

The cell membrane permits the passage of some substances, but not others, so is termed semipermeable. The relative permeability depends upon the ion, chloride being the most permeant ion. The H^+ hydrogen (a thin layer of glass) in pH electrodes is a perfect semipermeable membrane (i.e. does not allow passage of any solute molecules, but allows free passage of solvent).

Gibbs–Donnan equilibrium

Electrical and concentration gradients influence the movement of ions. The Gibbs–Donnan equilibrium states that both sides of a membrane are electrically neutral:

Distribution of ions across the cell membrane		
Component	**Outside**	**Inside**
K^+ (mmol/L)	4.5	140 (varies with cell type)
Na^+ (mmol/L)	140	10
Ca^{2+} total (mmol/L)	3	1
Ca^{2+} free	1 (μmol/L)	100 (nmol/L)
Cl^- (mmol/L)	110	3
HCO_3^- (mmol/L)	24	10
pH	7.35	7
amino acids, proteins	10	120

Fig. 3.10 Distribution of ions across the cell membrane.

[cation inside] = [anion inside]

[cation outside] = [anion outside]

The product of diffusible ions is equal on both sides:

[diffusible cations outside] × [diffusible anions outside] = [diffusible cations inside] × [diffusible anions inside]

Pores, channels, and pumps

The sodium pump reaches a steady state. Where there are fixed concentrations of ions on either side of the membrane. This is not in equilibrium as there is an unequal distribution of ions, with the inside being negative with respect to the outside. Energy input is required to form this distribution.

Transport across the membrane
Passive diffusion

Passive diffusion is the free movement of molecules across a membrane down a concentration gradient. No energy is required and it will continue until equilibrium is reached. It is directly proportional to the ion gradient, hydrostatic pressure, and electrical potential and can be summarized by Fick's law of diffusion:

flux = D × Area × Δ conc
Where D= diffusion constant, A= membrane area and Δ conc= concentration gradient

- Saturation does not occur as no binding sites are involved.
- Fick's law does not account for the dissolution of molecules in the lipid membrane.
- Increasing hydrophobicity increases passage through the membrane.
- Gated ion channels operate by simple diffusion (i.e. a gated channel or voltage receptor allows ions to diffuse freely when a receptor binding causes the channel to open.)

Facilitated diffusion

This is also called facilitated transport and occurs when a molecule moves down the concentration gradient via a receptor until equilibrium is achieved with no input of energy being required. This transport shows Michaelis–Menten kinetics (Fig. 3.11):

- Substrate specificity or selectivity, affinity for a particular ligand (measured as K_L).
- Saturability of ligand binding (B_{max}).
- Transferability (T_{max}), the maximum rate of molecule transfer across the membrane.
- Inhibition (e.g. transport of glucose into erythrocytes.)

If the molecule is charged, the electrical potential across the membrane must be accounted for (e.g. Ca^{2+}/Na^+ antiport system in the plasma membrane).

Active transport

Active transport moves molecules against an electrochemical or concentration gradient using energy supplied by the hydrolysis of adenosine triphosphate (ATP). It is sensitive to inhibitors that stop ATP synthesis (e.g. cyanide). It shows Michaelis kinetics, and uses up to half of the cell's energy. Primary active transport is principally linked to maintaining the intracellular and plasma sodium and potassium concentrations (e.g. sodium pump).

Secondary active transport links the Na^+/K^+ ATPase to a second transporter, which is not itself energy dependent. The second transporter transports molecules with or against a concentration or electrical gradient.

Symport transport is where the transported and co-transported molecule both move in the same direction, whereas antiport transport is where the molecules move in opposite directions (e.g. small intestine

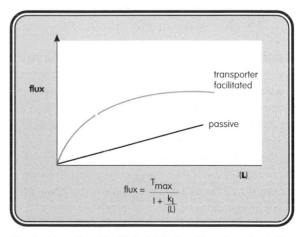

Fig. 3.11 Kinetics of facilitated diffusion. (T_{max}, transferability; k_L, affinity for ligand; [L], concentration of ligand.)

absorption of glucose and amino acids is linked to sodium transport, Fig. 3.12).

Summary of types of transport
In summary:
- Passive diffusion is via selective pores.
- Facilitated diffusion and active transport both require specific carrier proteins.
- Active transport requires energy.

Transport mechanisms
Membrane transport proteins are responsible for transferring molecules, and act either as channels or carriers.

Ion channels
Ion channels are proteins that span the membrane and have central water-filled pores. The pores are specific (allowing either cations only or anions only through). Transport speed is greater than 10^6 ions/s, but always passive. Pores may also be gated, and open and close in response to membrane changes, for example:
- Voltage-gated channels—respond to voltage changes in membrane potential.
- Ligand-gated channels—respond to binding with molecules.
- Mechanical-gated channels—respond to mechanical stimulation.

The potassium channel is the most common ion channel. It opens non-specifically, with the leakage of potassium through these channels being critical to the membrane potential. Defects or damage can cause muscular dysfunction (e.g. periodic paralysis).

Carrier proteins
These are used to enable polar and ionic molecules to pass through the membrane by passive and facilitated diffusion. Transport is hundreds of times slower than via ion channels. They are highly specific, and the specific binding to the carrier protein enables either the transporter to undergo a structural change, which produces a channel for the molecule to pass through, or alternately the carrier molecule flips to the other side of the bilayer, and releases the bound ion. Carrier proteins can become saturated, limiting the rate of transport. Uniports transport single molecules across

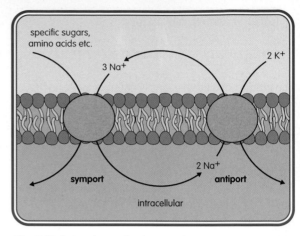

Fig. 3.12 Secondary active transport.

the membrane. Coupled transporters transport molecules across the membrane by simultaneous transfer of another molecule:
- Symports are coupled transporters transferring both molecules in the same direction.
- Antiports transfer the molecules in opposite directions to each other.

Different cells have different carrier cell populations, so differing permeabilities.

Glucose transporter
Most cells transfer glucose by passive diffusion through antiports as the concentration of glucose is greater outside the cell. In the intestine and kidney some cells are required to uptake glucose from low extracellular concentrations, and this is done via symports co-transporting sodium.

Active transporters
Active transporters are carrier proteins that are linked to a source of energy, such as ATP or an ionic gradient.

Sodium pump
The sodium pump is an example of an active transporter. It is a tetramer of two glycosylated α subunits and two non-glycosylated β subunits (Fig. 3.13). The α subunit is the catalytic unit, and has binding sites for sodium and ATP on its intracellular surface and potassium on its extracellular surface.

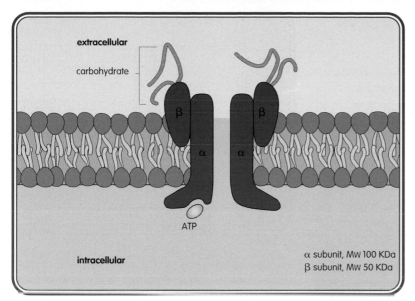

extracellular

carbohydrate

β

β

α

α

ATP

intracellular

α subunit, Mw 100 KDa
β subunit, Mw 50 KDa

Fig. 3.13 Structure of the sodium pump.

Binding of sodium causes phosphorylation of the cytoplasmic side and a conformational change, which transfers the sodium outside the cell. Binding of potassium causes dephosphorylation, so the subunit returns to its original state, transferring the potassium inside the cell simultaneously (Fig. 3.14). The biochemical name for the sodium pump is sodium/potassium (Na^+/K^+) ATPase. A steady state is reached when there is electroneutrality (i.e. any microscopic region has equal positive and negative charges, Fig. 3.15).

Functions of the sodium pump are as follows:

- Maintaining the intracellular sodium concentration at a low level.
- Regulation of intracellular K^+ concentration controls cell volume and osmolarity, thus the sodium pump regulates cell volume.
- Providing a sodium gradient as an energy source for co-transport, which is used by many body processes (e.g. sodium–hydrogen exchanger). If the sodium pump fails, many other processes in the cell fail. This accounts for the toxicity of digitalis in overdose since the cardiac glycosides are inhibitors of the sodium pump.
- Generation of membrane potential. Potassium leaks out of the cell down the steep concentration gradient, causing the inside of the cell to be negatively charged compared with the outside.

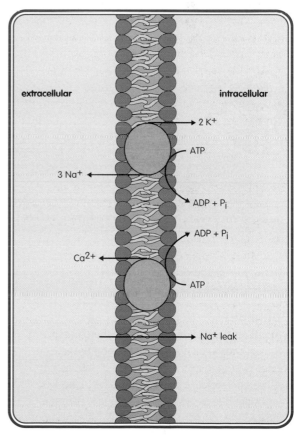

extracellular   intracellular

2 K^+

ATP

3 Na^+

ADP + P_i

ADP + P_i

Ca^{2+}

ATP

Na^+ leak

Fig. 3.14 Active transport by the sodium pump and calcium pump. (ADP, adenosine diphosphate; ATP, adenosine triphosphate; P_i, inorganic phosphate.)

37

Summary of types of transporter molecule

In summary:

- All transport molecules are proteins.
- Ion channels span the membrane, never require energy, and transport only with the gradient.
- Carrier proteins bind molecules, may be linked to an energy source, and can transport with or against a gradient.

A common error in exams is to confuse the sodium pump with an ion channel. It is not an ion channel as the sodium pump is linked to an energy source, has binding sites, and transports molecules against their concentration gradient.

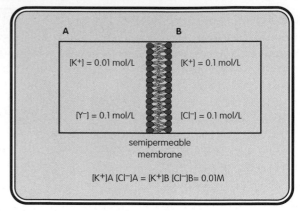

$$[K^+]A \ [Cl^-]A = [K^+]B \ [Cl^-]B = 0.01M$$

Fig. 3.15 This example shows two compartments separated by a semipermeable membrane, which is permeable to H_2O, K^+, and Cl^-, but impermeable to Y^-. K^+ and Cl^- diffuse across the membrane until they are in equilibrium, as shown by the Gibbs–Donnan equation, which holds for any univalent cation and anion in equilibrium between two chambers. (There is no $[Cl^-]$ in compartment A due to the impermeable anions $[Y^-]$ attracting anions $[K^+]$, so at equilibrium all the Cl^- has moved into compatment B.)

- Define concentration, moles, osmosis, osmoles, and the normal plasma osmolarity.
- Describe the distribution of ions across the plasma membrane and maintenance of ion gradients.
- Discuss the three major types of membrane transport—passive, facilitated, and active.
- Discuss the difference between channels and carriers.
- Describe the mechanism of action (related to its structure) of the sodium pump.

MEMBRANE POTENTIAL

Definition

A membrane potential is defined by the difference in electrical charge on each side of a membrane. The electric charge results from unequal distribution of positive and negative ions on each side of the membrane due to active pumping and/or passive diffusion. The membrane potential (E_m) is very important in the functioning of excitable cells, especially nerve and muscle cells. These cells use the opening of gated channels, which allows ion flow, to cause a change in their membrane potential. There are three major types of gated channels in excitable cells:

- Voltage-gated channels (e.g. voltage-gated sodium channels used in action potential generation).
- Chemically gated channels (e.g. acetylcholine receptor channels in neuromuscular transmission).
- Mechanical receptors (e.g. touch receptor channels in sensory neurons).

Maintenance of membrane potential
Gibbs–Donnan effect and Nernst equation

The Gibbs–Donnan effect is an uneven distribution of ions across a membrane due to a higher protein concentration on one side.

This should not be confused with the Gibbs-Donnan equilibruim where also the product of diffusible ions is equal on both sides, but differs in that both sides of the membrance are electrically neutral. The membrane must be permeable to water and ions, but impermeable to protein. Proteins are anions, so will attract diffusible cations, causing a potential across the membrane, the protein side being negative (Fig. 3.16).

The product of diffusible ions on either side is equal. More diffusible ions occur on the protein side due to attrachtional of the negative protein and contribute to the oncotic pressure with the protein. For example plasma proteins contribute 9 mmHg of the total plasma oncotic pressure (16 mmHg), the other 7 mmHg being due to uneven distribution of diffusible ions.

The electrical potential across the membrane at equilibrium is equal to the equilibrium potential of each ion.

- Equilibrium occurs when the electrical and concentration gradients across the membrane balance each other.
- The membrane potential at equilibrium of a given ion is given by the Nernst equation:

$$E = \frac{RT}{zF} \times \frac{\text{Ln } C_{out}}{C_{in}}$$

where E is the equilibrium potential, R is the gas constant, T is absolute temperature, z is valency, and F is Faraday's constant. C_{out} = given ion concentration outside the cell. C_{in} = given ion concentration inside the cell. Alternatively:

$$E = 61.\log_{10}\frac{C_{out}}{C_{in}} \text{ at } 37°C$$

Thus at equilibrium:

$$E(Na^+) = E(Cl^-)$$

The Donnan ratio (r) is:

$$\frac{Na^+_A}{Na^+_B} = \frac{Cl^-_B}{Cl^-_A} = r$$

Where A=protein side, and B is otherside (fig. 3.16).

- The Donnan excess (e) is the excess diffusible ions, and contributes to the osmotic pressure difference across the membrane. It is calculated as follows.

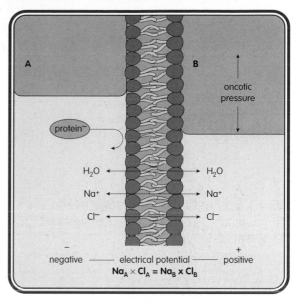

Fig. 3.16 Gibbs–Donnan effect. The equation expresses the Donnan excess, which contributes to osmotic pressure difference across the membrane.

The products of diffusible ions are equal on both sides:

$$Na^+_A \times Cl^-_A = Na^+_B \times Cl^-_B$$

Electroneutrality means the net charge of a solution is 0:

$$Na^+_A = Cl^-_A + Protein_A^-$$

$$Na^+_B = Cl^-_B$$

Thus:

$$Na^+_A \times Cl^-_A = [Na^+_B]^2 = [Cl^-_B]^2$$

The sum of the sides of a rectangle is greater than the sum of the sides of a square of the same area thus:

$$Na^+_A + Cl^-_A > Na^+_B + Cl^-_B$$

$$Na^+_A + Cl^-_A = Na^+_B + Cl^-_B + e$$

Where e = donnan excess

The volumes of each compartment need to be fixed for a Gibbs–Donnan distribution. The electrical potential of compartment B is balanced by hydrostatic pressure in compartment B, which prevents all the solution moving into compartment A.

The Gibbs–Donnan distribution occurs across capillary cell walls, but does not cause cell membrane potential as there is no Donnan ratio.

The constant field equation formed by Goldman and Hodgkin uses sodium and potassium permeabilities to estimate the cell membrane potential (E_m):

$$cm = -61 \log \frac{[K^+]_{in} + b[Na^+]_{in}}{[K^+]_{out} + b[Na^+]_{out}} \ [mV]$$

where b is permeability of Na (P_{Na})/permeability of K (P_K). Notice that if $b = 0$, this equation becomes the Nernst equation.

Muscle and nerve cells increase P_{Na} when activated, thus b increases from 1/100 to 10. Potassium permeability of nerve and muscle cells is hundreds of times higher than that of non-excitable cells, resulting in high resting potentials. Sodium permeability varies little between cells.

Potassium ion effect on membrane potential

The cell membrane is most permeable to potassium ions, which constantly leak through potassium ion channels. The cell has fixed negatively charged intracellular organic molecules that must be balanced by cations. This balance is largely achieved by potassium, as sodium concentration is too low inside the cell. The sodium pump moves potassium in, and ion channels allow potassium to leak out. Potassium approaches an equilibrium with:

- Electrical forces attracting it in to balance intracellular anions.
- The concentration gradient across the membrane causing it to move back out.

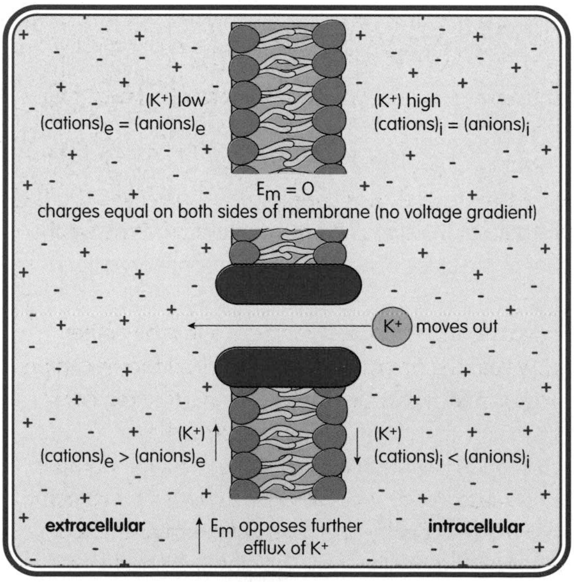

Thus the electrical potential across the cell is proportional to the concentration gradient of potassium across the membrane (Fig. 3.17).

When the electrochemical gradient is zero, the voltage difference across the membrane balances the gradient, and this is the resting potential of the cell, which can be calculated by the Nernst equation. Resting potential can vary from −20 mV to −200 mV, with the inside of the cell being negatively charged with respect to the outside. Other ions may influence the resting potential, their contribution being related to how readily they permeate the cell membrane. Increasing the membrane permeability of an ion drives the membrane potential towards that ion's equilibrium value.

Action potentials

An action potential is a rapid, transient, self-perpetuating electrical excitation of the membrane:

- Depolarization means the E_m becomes less negative, so there is a decrease in the potential difference.
- Hyperpolarization means that the potential difference increases in magnitude, by increasing the relative negative charge inside the cell.

Fig. 3.17 Role of potassium in generating the cell membrane potential. (E_m, membrane potential), e=extracellular, i=intracelluar.

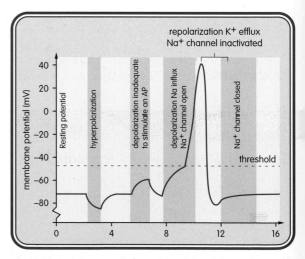

Fig. 3.18 Generation of an action potential.

Depolarization is the stimulus for the action potential (Fig. 3.18). Voltage-gated sodium channels produce the action potential, by opening in response to initial depolarization.

A threshold rise in the membrane potential must be reached before the action potential occurs. Opening of the voltage-gated channels at threshold EM, allows more sodium to enter the cell, causing further depolarization. The magnitude and duration of the action potential are fixed and do not vary with the magnitude and duration of the initial stimulus. When the driving force for sodium flow reaches zero the channels become inactivated. The channels are now refractory and are unable to open again until the cell repolarizes, so reaching its original resting potential. Return to the resting potential is caused by efflux of potassium.

The local circuit hypothesis states that propagation occurs where the current flows along the membrane, generating areas of local depolarization, this depolarization produces action potentials in areas ahead (Fig. 3.19). Propagation is unidirectional, as regions that have just been excited are refractory. The thousands of channels summate to create a current across the membrane that can be measured with a microelectrode.

Action potentials function in the body as:
- Communication mechanisms for electrical signals along nerve and muscle cells.
- Pathways for coordinated activity.
- Respiratory and behavioural patterns (spontaneous action potentials).

See *Crash Course, Nervous System & Special Senses* and *Crash Course, Musculoskeletal System* for further details.

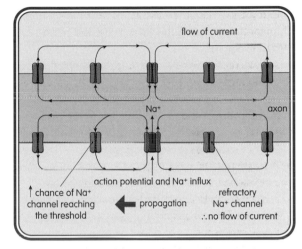

Fig. 3.19 Propagation of the action potential, illustrating the local circuit hypothesis.

- **Define a membrane potential.**
- **Calculate an ion's membrane potential using the Nernst equation.**
- **Describe the Gibbs–Donnan effect due to non-diffusible protein causing uneven ion distribution.**
- **Define an action potential.**
- **Discuss the production and propagation of an action potential.**

RECEPTORS

Concepts of transmembrane signalling
Mechanisms to signal from extracellular to intracellular are necessary

Only certain lipid-soluble molecules can cross the cell membrane directly (e.g. steroid hormones); other molecules transfer their signal by binding cell surface receptors. Signal transduction has been shown to be a universal path through which cells are directed to divide, differentiate to express non-replicative proteins, increase cell activity, degranulate and many other activities. The pathway begins at cell surface receptors and ends in the nucleus with proteins that regulate gene expression. The paths are formed by interconnecting proteins, which can amplify, dampen, or process signals before passing them downstream. There is economy of the effector system as there are many ligands and receptors, but few second messengers, which in turn can have many effects on cell function. Transduction enables responses to be made to external factors governing cell activity.

There is integration of a variety of signals, so before a decision is made the cell will assess its cellular neighbours, environment, substratum contact, and the presence of growth factors and hormones. When the pathway malfunctions, the cell may multiply uncontrollably, and this may result in a carcinoma. Oncogenes are part of the signalling path.

Definitions

Important definitions include the following:

- Cell surface receptors are specific proteins that bind a signalling molecule and convert this binding into intracellular signals, which alter the cell's behaviour.
- A ligand is a molecule that binds the receptor, and is the first messenger.
- A hormone is a molecule produced by an endocrine cell, that is released into the bloodstream and acts on specific receptors. Steroid hormones are synthesized from cholesterol and are hydrophobic.
- The second-messenger system is a set of intracellular molecules that are activated by cell surface receptors and affect cell function, producing a physiological response e.g. AMP, GMP, DAG, PIP_α.

The three mechanisms of cell signalling to surface receptors are:

- Endocrine.
- Paracrine.
- Autocrine.

The same molecules and receptors may be used in all three mechanisms (Fig. 3.20).

Types of receptor

Ionotropic receptors

These receptors are linked to an ion channel and are made of multimeric proteins of about 250 000 Da. They are predominantly found in the nervous system, and their signalling is very fast (e.g. nicotinic acetylcholine receptor) which has five subunits (2α, β, γ, δ) (Fig. 3.21).

Tyrosine kinase (TK) receptors

These are catalytic receptors that signal directly to the cell (Fig. 3.22). There are four classes and these are illustrated in Fig. 3.23. TK phosphorylates target proteins (Fig. 3.24), often including its own cytoplasmic tail in a process known as 'autophosphorylation'. Cytoplasmic proteins, which are often enzymes, bind to activated TK through a

Fig. 3.20 The three mechanisms of cell signalling.

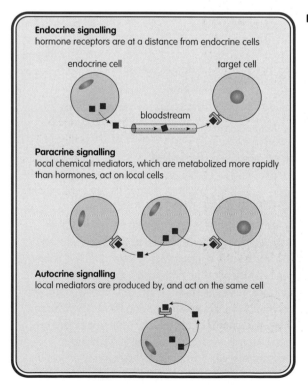

Endocrine signalling
hormone receptors are at a distance from endocrine cells

endocrine cell   target cell

bloodstream

Paracrine signalling
local chemical mediators, which are metabolized more rapidly than hormones, act on local cells

Autocrine signalling
local mediators are produced by, and act on the same cell

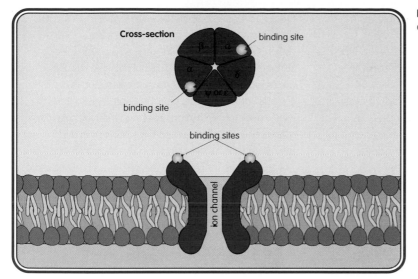

Fig. 3.21 Structure of the nicotinic acetylcholine receptor.

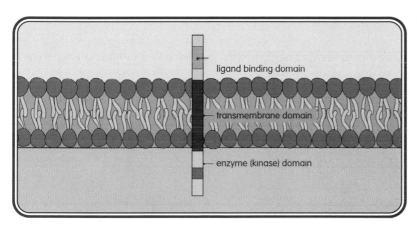

Fig. 3.22 Structure of the TK receptor.

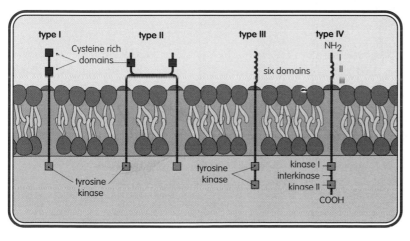

Fig. 3.23 The four classes of TK receptor. All these receptors have tyrosine kinase activity and SH$_2$ binding domains on their cytoplasmic portions. The receptors chain differences are between their ligand binding domains.

common domain, the SH2 domain. Examples of TK receptors are:

- Epidermal growth factor (EGF) receptor—a type I TK receptor; its ligands are EGF, tumour growth factor (TGF) α, and heparin binding EGF, which all have a similar core structure. In inflammatory disease such as pancreatitis there may be upregulation of EGF receptors, which bind TGF α that can lead to abnormal growth and possibly carcinoma.
- Insulin growth factor (IGF) I receptor—a type II TK receptor.
- Fibroblast growth factor (FGF) receptors—all type IV TK receptors. There are four FGF receptors, which bind the seven FGF ligands. FGF is important in angiogenesis, and abnormalities of FGF and the FGF receptor are seen in some carcinomas (e.g. pancreatic), encouraging both paracrine and autocrine proliferation.

Metabotropic receptors (G-protein coupled)

These receptors all have a common structural feature, a region that spans the membrane seven times (Fig. 3.25). Some receptors are composed of multiple subunits and are activated by dissociation of these subunits. Metabotropic receptors activate G-proteins, a 2nd messenger family that are bound to the inner plasma membrane. When activated G-proteins bind and hydrolyse GTP, functioning like a binary switch (Fig. 3.26). The *ras* protein (encoded by an oncogene) belongs to a subset of G-proteins. Activated G-proteins subsequently activate intracellular second-messenger pathways, for example:

- Cyclic adenosine monophosphate (cAMP) (Fig. 3.27).
- Calcium (directly by opening of calcium channels in the plasma membrane, or indirectly by the inositol lipid pathways).
- Inositol lipid pathways (Fig. 3.28).

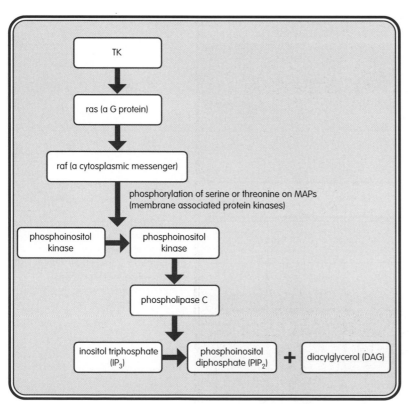

Fig. 3.24 TK signal transduction, showing phosphorylation path of target proteins.

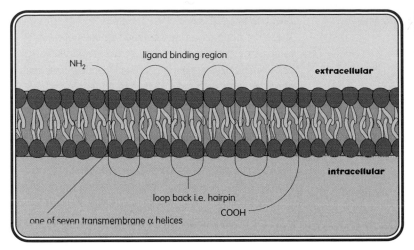

Fig. 3.25 Structure of a metabotropic receptor.

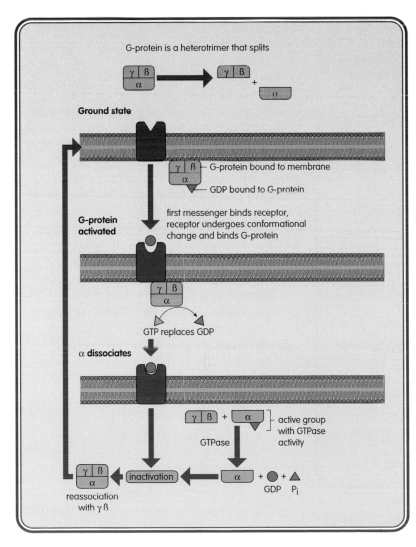

Fig. 3.26 Activation of G-proteins. (GDP, guanosine diphosphate; GTP, guanosine triphosphate; P_i, inorganic phosphate.)

Different G-proteins activate different pathways, for example:

- G_s increases cAMP (Fig. 3.27).
- G_i decreases cAMP.
- G_q activates the inositol lipid pathway.

An example of a metabotropic receptor is the β-adrenergic receptor.

The TK receptor is commonly mistaken for a metabotrophic receptor as it has a G-protein linked transduction mechanism. However, it is not a metabotropic receptor as it does not have a seven-pass membrane structure.

Steroid receptors

These are not membrane bound receptors, but soluble cytoplasmic proteins (Fig. 3.28). Steroid receptors bind water-insoluble steroid, retinoid, and thyroid hormones, which pass through the lipid membrane easily and are metabolized more slowly when released into the bloodstream than are hydrophilic molecules.

Once activated, the receptors may or may not dimerise before binding specific nucleotide sequences on the DNA, so regulating the transcription of specific genes. The product of the gene may in turn regulate the transcription of further genes, termed the secondary response. The testosterone receptor is a steroid receptor.

Receptors and drugs

Many drugs produce their pharmacological effect by acting on cell surface receptors. The effect produced depends upon whether the drug acts as an agonist or antagonist:

- Agonists are molecules that activate receptors and may be pharmacological or physical agents.
- Antagonists are molecules that bind receptors, do not activate them; they block the receptor's ligand from binding, so preventing the ligand's action.

Reversible antagonists, also called competitive antagonists, compete with the ligand for the receptor. They can be reversed by increasing the concentration of agonist. Irreversible antagonists cannot be removed from the receptor; thus they reduce the effective number of receptors and cannot be reversed by increasing the agonist concentration.

The specificity of a drug reflects its ability to combine with one receptor type. The desired action of a drug is to combine with a specific receptor in the targetted tissue. Adverse effects may be caused by non-specific binding to other receptor types, or by binding with the desired receptor, but in a different tissue.

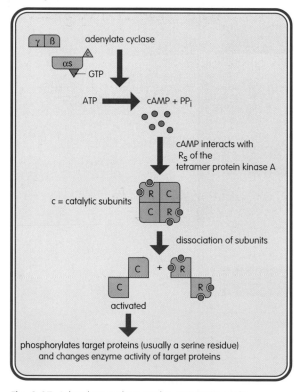

Fig. 3.27 Adenylate cyclase pathway (cAMP, cyclic adenosine monophosphate; ATP, adenosine triphosphate; C, catalytic subunits; GTP, guanosine triphosphate; PP$_i$, pyrophosphate; R, regulatory subunits).

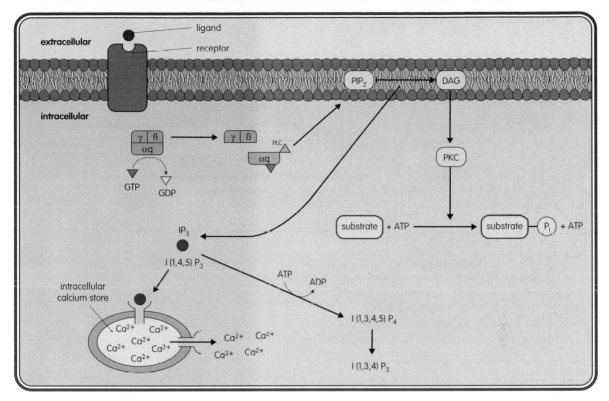

Fig. 3.28 Inositol phospholipid signalling pathway (PLC, phospholipase c; GTP, guanosine triphosphate; ADP, guanosine monophosphate; PIP$_2$, phosphoinositol diphosphate; DAG, diacylglycerol; PKC, phosphokinase C; P$_i$, inorganic phosphate; IP$_3$, inositol triphosphate; Ca^{2+}, calcium ions).

Fig. 3.29 Structure of a steroid receptor.

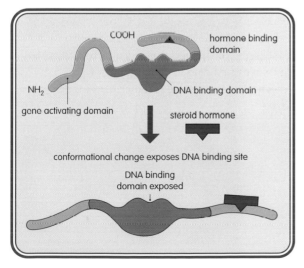

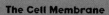

- Name the functions of transmembrane signalling mechanisms—list at least four.
- Define a cell surface receptor, ligand, hormone, and second-messenger system.
- Define autocrine, paracrine, and endocrine signalling.
- Describe the structure and function of ionotropic, TK, metabotropic, and steroid receptors.
- Discuss the effects of drugs acting as receptor agonists or antagonists.
- Draw a diagram to show the CAMP and IP_3 based 2nd messenger/transduction pathways.

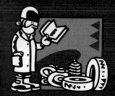

4. The Working Cell

CYTOSKELETON AND CELL MOTILITY

Concepts

The cytoskeleton is composed of filamentous proteins in the cytosol. The cytoskeleton's major functions are:

- Determining cell shape (mechanical).
- Organelle anchoring and polarity determination.
- Motility (and migration).
- Anchoring of the cell to external structures.
- Metabolic functions.
- Cell division spindle for separating duplicated chromatids into separate cells.

Shape determination is very important, and is often fundamental to cell functioning (e.g. microvilli increase the absorption area of intestinal cells).

Components of the cytoskeleton

Actin

A microfilament is composed of actin and is 6–7 nm wide. The subunit, G-actin, is globular, and at least six kinds are known. The filament, F-actin, is formed by the polymerization of G-actin subunits (Fig. 4.1). Each G-actin has defined polarity, polymerizing head to tail, so F-actin also has defined polarity. Polymerization and depolymerization of fibres are closely regulated by the cell.

Actin is the product of different genes in muscle and non-muscle cells, so the properties of these two types of actin differ. Minor amino acid differences between muscle and non-muscle actins may allow them to bind

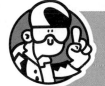

The functions of the cytoskeleton are a common topic for exam questions; remember to give examples for full marks and do not just name the functions.

different proteins and account for their different functions. Actin has a contractile function in muscle cells. In non-muscle cells, actin:

- Maintains microvilli structure.
- Forms part of the terminal web, which lies beneath microvilli and desmosomes.
- Causes movement of macrophages by gel–sol transition of the actin network.
- Causes movement of fibroblasts and nerve growth cones by controlled polymerization and rearrangement of actin filaments.

There are various actin-binding proteins, which are also called microfilament accessory proteins (Fig. 4.2). These cause changes in the molecular forms of actin, and can be classified into four groups according to their functions:

- They can affect actin–myosin interactions—these actin-binding proteins are found in all cells and regulate actin and myosin head binding and may cause actin filaments to move. This group includes

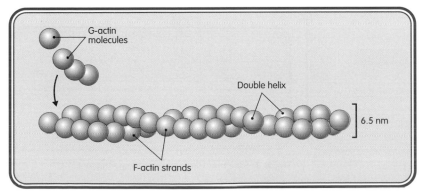

Fig. 4.1 Structure of a microfilament.

troponin in striated muscle, which is replaced by calmodulin in non-striated cells, and smooth muscle.

- They can regulate polymerization of G-actin to F-actin—for example gelsolin will polymerize or depolymerize actin depending upon the calcium concentration, capping proteins prevent loss or addition to actin, profilin prevents polymerization of actin.
- They can crosslink F-actin filaments—for example spectrin, fodrin, and filamin crosslink adjacent actin fibres, while fimbrin, fascin, and villin crosslink actin to form parallel fibres.
- They can mediate attachment of actin filaments to the plasma membrane—this group includes proteins that link actin to the cell membrane (e.g. α-actinin, β-actinin, talin, and vinculin).

In non-muscle cells, microfilament accessory proteins serve both structural and contractile functions.

Intermediate filaments

Intermediate filaments are 8–11 nm wide and are also polymers, but are more stable than microfilaments and microtubules (Fig. 4.3). Intermediate filaments are always filaments at physiological pH and ionic concentrations, whereas microfilaments and tubules exist as both monomers and filaments under physiological conditions. Intermediate filaments are

thought to be the major structural determinants in cells. There are many varieties, for example:

- Cytokeratins—these are typically expressed in the epithelium. Ten cytokeratins are specific to 'hard' tissues (e.g. nail and hair). Approximately 20 cytokeratins are found more generally in epithelia lining internal body cavities.
- Neurofilaments—these are found in neuron axons. They may account for the strength and rigidity of the axon.
- Glial fibrillary acidic protein (GFAP)—this is found in glial cells surrounding neurons.
- Vimentin—this is expressed in mesenchymal cells such as fibroblasts, and in endothelial cells. These fibres often end at the nuclear membrane and desmosomes. They are closely associated with microtubules, and form cages around lipid droplets in adipose tissue.
- Desmin—this is found predominantly in muscle cells. It forms an interconnecting network perpendicular to the long axis of the cell. Desmin fibres anchor and orientate the Z bands in myofibrils, thus generating the striated pattern.

Rapidly growing cells and myelin-producing glial cells do not have intermediate filaments. Cells usually contain only one type of intermediate filament.

Microtubules

Microtubules are hollow tubules and are 25 nm wide (Fig. 4.4). Tubulin is a dimeric structural unit (αβ dimer). Microtubules are formed from filaments, which in turn are formed from dimers by polymerization. Tubulin and the structures it forms are polar.

Colchicine and the vinca alkaloids depolymerize microtubules. Microtubules form the cell division spindle; thus colchicine and vincristine disassemble this structure and can be used as anticancer agents.

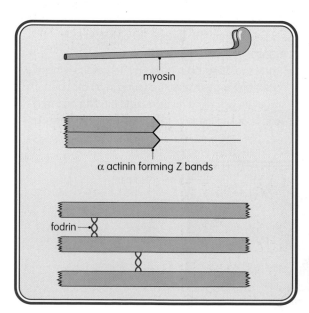

Fig. 4.2 Examples of actin-binding proteins.

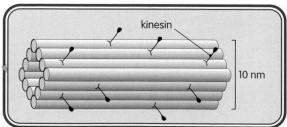

Fig. 4.3 Structure of an intermediate filament.

Microtubules are strong and all cells have microtubules, except for mature erythrocytes; they are abundant in neurons.

There are many microtubule associated proteins (MAPs), which:

- Have specific associations with the tubulin, with different microtubules containing different MAPs.
- Can accelerate the polymerization of tubulin and form armlike processes, which can crosslink adjacent microtubules.
- In the nerve axon are called Tau (τ).

Different MAPs include:

- Kinesin, which is bound to microtubules and can transport vesicles along the microtubule in the presence of adenosine triphosphate (ATP). Kinesin moves in an antegrade direction (i.e. from the cell body to the axon terminal).
- MAP1C, which is associated with ATP-powered transport and moves in a retrograde direction.
- Dynein, which functions to enable microtubule sliding movement.

- The centrioles, which assemble microtubules into a spindle during cell division.

Microtubules can form cilia and flagella, both of which move via ATP-powered dynein arm linkage. Cilia are found in the respiratory tract and fallopian tube whereas flagella are found on sperm. Microtubules also act as a track for transporting small vesicles within the cytoplasm and contribute to cell polarity.

Myosin

Myosin is composed of two heavy chains and four light chains (Fig. 4.5). The two essential light chains have ATPase action. The two regulatory light chains determine the binding of calmodulin to myosin. Myosin in muscle and non-muscle cells varies in its amino acid sequence. Actin and myosin interact to produce contraction, which is regulated by:

- Troponin in skeletal muscle.
- Calmodulin in non-muscle cells.

See *Crash Course, Musculoskeletal System* for further details.

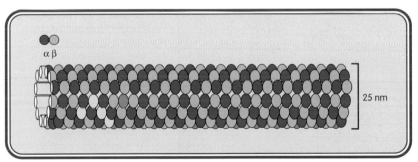

Fig. 4.4 Structure of a microtubule. There are normally 12–13 tubulin units per turn in the assembled microtubule. (Adapted with permission from *Molecular Biology of the Cell 3e*, by B. Alberts, D. Bray, J. Lewis, M. Raff, K. Roberts and J. D. Watson, Garland Publishing, 1994.)

α β

25 nm

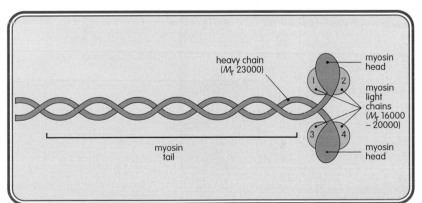

Fig. 4.5 Structure of myosin.(M_r, relative molecular mass.)

heavy chain (M_r 23000)

myosin head

myosin light chains (M_r 16000 – 20000)

myosin tail

myosin head

Examples of cytoskeletal function

Erythrocyte cytoskeleton

Erythrocytes have a very rigid but deformable shape. The cytoskeleton is atypically distributed, being present in only a thin strip below the cell membrane. Patients with hereditary spherocytosis and elliptocytosis produce smaller amounts or defective spectrin, so their erythrocytes are less deformable, lose their biconcave shape, and become trapped in the circulation (see *Crash Course, Immune, Blood, and Lymphatic Systems*).

Cilia

Cilia are formed of a 9+2 arrangement of microtubules with a basal body (Fig. 4.6). Dynein arms connect microtubule pairs, and the sliding mechanism enables the cilia to bend (see Fig. 1.11).

Intestinal epithelium

Absorption is increased by microvillious projections which increase intestinal surface area (Fig. 4.7).

Axonal transport

Kinesins and MAP1C transport materials along axons, each moving in a different direction. Transport is normally at a rate of 25 mm/day (Fig. 4.8).

Muscle contraction

In skeletal muscle, the arrangement of parallel actin and myosin into sarcomeres allows maximum efficiency of contraction. In smooth muscle, the contractile subunits resemble sarcomeres, but are not as organized. (See *Crash Course, Musculoskeletal System* for further details.)

Motility of phagocytes

Phagocyte motility is achieved by projecting a foot-like pseudopodia, with a gel/sol transition state at its tip. Transition from a gel phase, where the actin in the cytoskeleton is polymerized, allows the pseudopodia to creep along to a sol phase, where the actin is depolymerized.

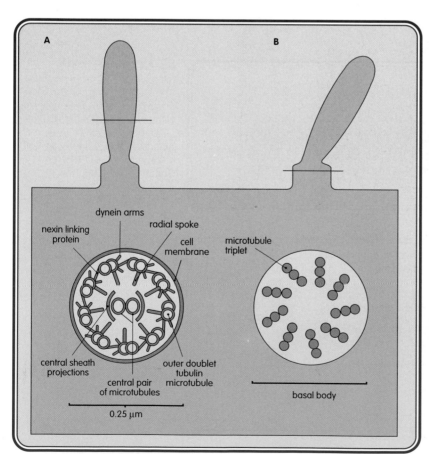

Fig. 4.6 Structure of (A) a cilium and (B) a basal body. Bending the dynein arms of one microtubule couplet links to the couplet in front, and these arm processes hydrolyse ATP, so the microtubules move relative to each other.

A

B

dynein arms

nexin linking protein

radial spoke

cell membrane

microtubule triplet

central sheath projections

central pair of microtubules

outer doublet tubulin microtubule

basal body

0.25 μm

Mitotic spindle

The spindle is a polar arrangement of microtubules across the equator of the cell. Chromosomes attach to the spindle via kinetochore protein, at their centromeres. Separation of chromatids occurs as the microtubules contract, pulling them to separate poles (see Chapter 5).

- Define the cytoskeleton.
- Describe the structure and function of actin, intermediate filaments, microtubules, and myosin.
- Describe the functions of the cytoskeleton with examples—list at least five.

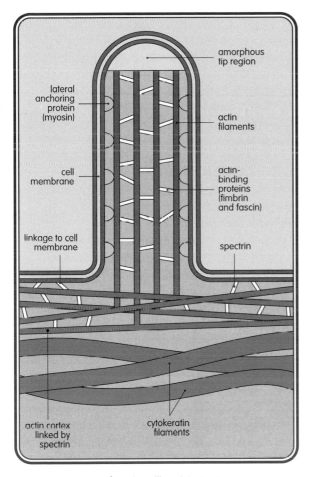

amorphous tip region

lateral anchoring protein (myosin)

cell membrane

linkage to cell membrane

actin cortex linked by spectrin

actin filaments

actin-binding proteins (fimbrin and fascin)

spectrin

cytokeratin filaments

Fig. 4.7 Structure of a microvillus. A helical arrangement of myosin molecules binds the actin bundle to the inner surface of the cell membrane.

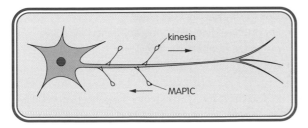

kinesin

MAP1C

Fig. 4.8 Kinesin and MAP1C transport materials along axons. Axoplasmic flow.

LYSOSOMES

Definition

A lysosome is a membrane-bound organelle that contains acid hydrolases capable of breaking down macromolecules (see Fig. 1.9).

Lysosomes:

- Were first discovered by de Duve.
- Have diameters ranging from 50 nm to 1 mm.
- Have a single membrane made up of a phospholipid bilayer that can selectively fuse with other membranes. At least 16 proteins are contained in the membrane, including a protein ATPase, which acidifies the lysosomal matrix to pH 4.5–5.5.

New lysosomes are derived from the Golgi complex. Most cells have hundreds of lysosomes, with phagocytic cells containing thousands. Erythrocytes do not contain any lysosomes. Newly synthesized lysosomes are called primary lysosomes. Secondary lysosomes are formed from fusion with a vesicle containing substrate.

Functions of lysosomes

Lysosome functions are:

- Autophagy—digestion of material of intracellular origin (i.e. fuses with vacuoles from inside the cell).
- Heterophagy—digestion of material of extracellular origin (i.e. fuses with vacuoles from outside the cell—pinocytic, endocytic, or phagocytic).

Endocytosis is uptake that can be specific (receptor-mediated endocytosis) or non-specific (pinocytosis). Pinocytosis is the non-specific uptake of extracellular molecules in proportion to their extracellular concentration. Phagocytosis is the internalization of membrane-bound molecules by expansion and engulfment; it is not a form of endocytosis.

The lysosome has hydrolytic enzymes, which catalyze the breakdown of macromolecules into component residues. If allowed to leak out, as in lytic cell death, the hydrolases homogenize tissue. The products are of low molecular mass and are transported across the lysosomal membrane by appropriate transport proteins. Over 60 different lysosomal enzymes have been identified, some of which are:

- Nucleases (e.g. acid RNase, acid DNase).
- Glycosidases (e.g. β-glucuronidase, hyaluronidase).

Be careful not to misread questions with the words lysozyme or lysosome. Lysozyme is a glycosidase enzyme, but is not normally found in the organelle, lysosome.

- Carbohydrate degradation enzymes (e.g. β-galactosidase, α-glucosidase).
- Proteases (e.g. cathepsins, collagenase).
- Phosphatases (e.g. acid phosphatase).
- Sulphatases (e.g. aryl sulphatase).
- Lipases.

Following synthesis in the rough endoplasmic reticulum (RER), lysosomal enzymes are modified by glycosylation in the RER lumen and covalent modification in the Golgi apparatus. Covalent modification includes phosphorylation of mannose groups to produce mannose-6-phosphate groups, which act as recognition markers and direct the enzymes to primary lysosomes.

Receptor-mediated endocytosis

Receptor-mediated endocytosis occurs when molecules that bind specific surface receptors are internalized (Fig. 4.9). This process was elucidated by Brian Goldstein, who studied the low-density lipoprotein (LDL) receptor, and for which he earned a Nobel prize. There are many functions provided by receptor-mediated endocytosis, examples are listed in Fig. 4.10.

Lysosomal storage diseases

These are disorders of lysosomal function and result in macromolecules becoming trapped inside the lysosome. The lysosome enlarges, causing the tissue to enlarge and resulting in pathological features. The causes of storage disorders are:

- Enzymatic—due to enzyme deficiency, defective enzymes, or absence of activator.
- Nonenzymatic—due to transporter defects.

Each disorder is rare, but together they affect 1 in 4800 live births. They are commonly fatal, but can be diagnosed prenatally. All show recessive inheritance, most being autosomal, except for two that are X-linked. Features leading to suspicion of a lysosomal storage disorder are:

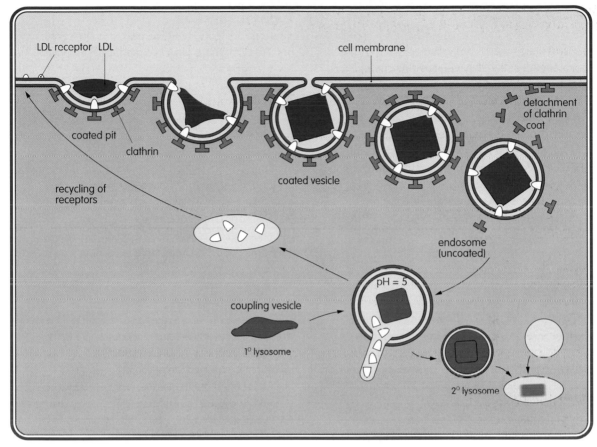

Fig. 4.9 Mechanism of receptor-mediated endocytosis. Clathrin is the coat protein that surrounds and internalises the pit. (LDL, low-density lipoprotein.)

Functions of receptor-mediated endocytosis	
Molecules taken up	**Function**
low-density lipoprotein (LDL)	transports of TAGs and cholesterol
transferrin	transports iron
insulin	affects cell metabolism
fibrin	removes injurious agents

Fig. 4.10 Functions of receptor-mediated endocytosis.

- Progressive neurological degeneration.
- Hepato (spleno) megaly.
- Skeletal dysplasia with or without short stature.
- Coarse facies.
- Eye changes (e.g. cherry red spot, corneal clouding).

Gaucher's disease

Gaucher's disease is the commonest lysosomal storage disorder (incidence 1 in 25 000 live births). Inheritance is autosomal recessive, with a high incidence seen in Ashkenazi Jews, who have a carrier frequency of 1 in 60. There is a deficiency of β-glucosidase, resulting in accumulation of its substrate glucocerebroside. The enzyme is coded on chromosome 1. There are allelic variants resulting in three major types of Gaucher's disease.

- Type I—adult type, non-neuronopathic.
- Type II—severe infantile, rare, neurological signs seen at three months, die by two years of age.
- Type III—subacute, neuronopathic, variable presentation from childhood to 70 years of age.

Treatment approaches for Gaucher's disease involve enzyme replacement therapy, bone marrow transplantation, and gene therapy.

Tay–Sachs disease

This is due to lack of the hexosaminidase A α chain, resulting in accumulation of ganglioside GM2. The hexosaminidase A α chain is coded on chromosome 15 position q22–25, and inheritance is autosomal recessive. There is an increased incidence in Ashkenazi Jews (carrier frequency is 1 in 25 compared with the UK general population carrier frequency of 1 in 250). Affected children are normal at birth, with symptoms beginning at 4–8 months of age, and death occurring by 3–4 years. Carrier screening is available, using an enzyme assay of the hexosaminidase system. Treatment is not yet available.

- ◦ **Define a lysosome.**
- ◦ **Name examples of lysosomal enzymes— list at least five.**
- ◦ **Discuss the difference between endocytosis, pinocytosis, and phagocytosis.**
- ◦ **Describe the receptor-mediated endocytosis pathway.**
- ◦ **Describe the salient features of lysosomal storage disorders.**

CELL SURFACE AND CELL ADHESION

Importance of cellular interaction and adhesion

Interactions between cells, and with the extracellular matrix (ECM), largely carry out a structural role, but are also important in cell migration, growth, immunological functions, permeability, cell recognition, tissue repair, differentiation, and embryogenesis.

Cells respond to components in the ECM by adherence to specific receptors. In epithelium there is little ECM, so cell–cell interactions also bear mechanical stresses.

Types of junction

Junctions are found between cells, and between cells and the ECM. There are three groups of cell junction, as listed in Fig. 4.11.

Tight junctions

All epithelia act as selectively permeable barriers, with tight junctions blocking diffusion of membrane proteins between apical (top) and basolateral (sides at the bottom) domains of the plasma membrane and sealing neighbouring cells together so that water-soluble molecules cannot leak between cells (Fig. 4.12). The ability to restrict ion passage increases logarithmically with the number of strands (e.g. small intestine tight junctions are 10 000 times more leaky than bladder tight junctions).

Anchoring junctions

Anchoring junctions are most abundant in cells under stress (e.g. cardiac muscle). They are made up of:
- Intracellular attachment proteins.
- Transmembrane linker glycoproteins.
- ECM or transmembrane linker glycoproteins on another cell (Fig. 4.13).

Anchoring junctions containing actin filament connections are called adherens junctions. Adherens cell–ECM junctions connect cell actin to ECM via focal contacts.

Types of cell junction	
Group	**Members**
occluding junctions	tight junctions
anchoring junctions	actin filament attachment sites: (adherens junctions) cell–cell (e.g. adhesion belts) cell–matrix (e.g. focal contacts) intermediate filament attachment sites: cell–cell (e.g. desmosomes) cell–matrix (e.g. hemidesmosomes)
communicating junctions	gap junctions chemical synapses

Fig. 4.11 Types of cell junction.

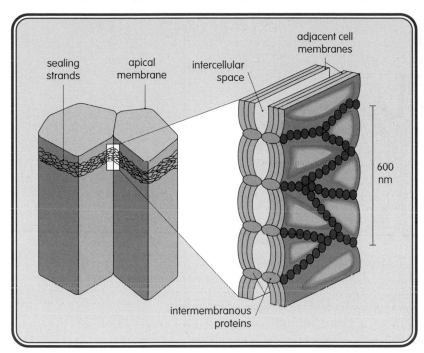

Fig. 4.12 Structure of a tight junction.

Adherens cell–cell junctions occur as streaklike attachments in non-epithelial cells and as continuous belts just below tight junctions in epithelial cells. The structure is the same as the ECM–cell junction. The membranes are held together by a Ca^{2+}-dependent mechanism mediated by cadherins. Actin bundles are linked into a network that lies parallel to the membrane. These adheren junctions with their attached actin bundles mediate neural tube formation in the embryo.

Desmosomes link intermediate filaments from cell to cell, and provide tensile strength (Fig. 4.14). Autoimmune disease against desmogleins causes pemphigus a blistering skin disorder.

Gap junctions

These are communicating junctions that allow inorganic ions carrying current and water-soluble molecules to pass directly from one cell to another, hence allowing electrical and metabolic cell coupling

Four α helices form a connexin. Six connexins form a connexon, the pore of which is formed from one α helix of each protein. Connexons of neighbouring cells align to form a continuous aqueous channel (Fig. 4.15). Molecules of up to 1300 D can pass through the 1.5 nm pore. Several

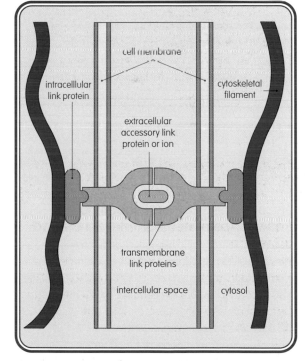

Fig. 4.13 General structure of an anchoring junction. Different (or multiple) link proteins and transmembrane proteins operate for the different classes of junction.

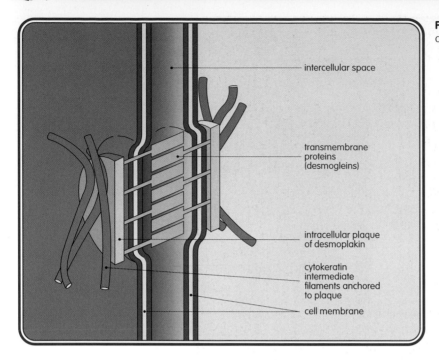

Fig. 4.14 Structure of a desmosome.

intercellular space

transmembrane proteins (desmogleins)

intracellular plaque of desmoplakin

cytokeratin intermediate filaments anchored to plaque

cell membrane

thousand connexons form a gap junction. Some pores are gated, with opening related to a three-dimensional change, which is often mediated via extracellular signals. Electrical coupling via gap junctions is important in:

- Peristalsis.
- Synchrony of heart contractions.
- Coordination of ciliated epithelium.

Gap junctions play a role in embryogenesis by allowing gradients of morphogens to form across blocks of cells.

Glycoproteins and cell labelling

Surface glycoproteins are important in cell recognition processes, with specific oligosaccharide chains allowing cells to recognize each other. Examples are:

- ABO blood groups.
- Major histocompatibility complex (MHC) antigens.

The ABO blood groups are determined by the carbohydrates (agglutinogens) found on the erythrocyte membrane. Antibodies to the agglutinogens not present on the host erythrocytes are contained in plasma. If a transfusion contains erythrocytes with agglutinogens that are not found on the recipient's

erythrocytes, the donor red blood cells will be agglutinated and then haemolysed (Fig. 4.16). Group O is the 'universal donor' and AB the 'universal recipient'.

The MHC codes for glycoproteins that are found on all of an individual's cells (except erythrocytes), and this mechanism helps host immunity distinguish between 'self' and 'foreign' cells (see *Crash Course Immune, Blood, and Lymphatic Systems*).

Adhesion molecules

There are four major cell adhesion molecule families (Fig. 4.17):

- Cadherins.
- Immunoglobulin superfamily.
- Selectins.
- Integrins.

Cadherins

The cadherins are single-pass glycoproteins that mediate communication and adhesion (Fig. 4.18). There are two homophilic binding sites. Homophilic binding is where two cells with the same protein adhere to each other through the same protein (i.e. the protein is both the ligand and the receptor and must therefore have two

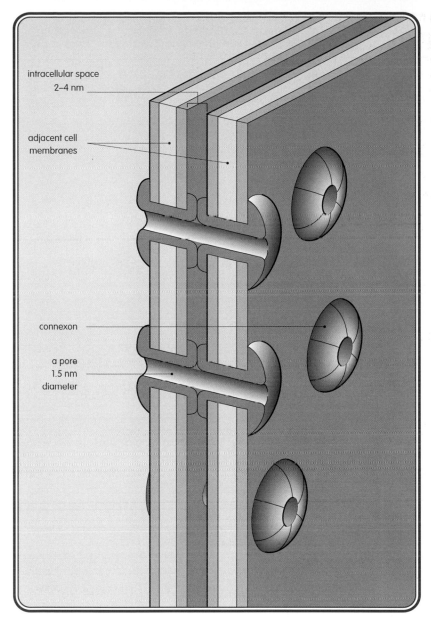

Fig. 4.15 Structure of part of a gap junction. Each junction consists of several hundred pores, which are aligned on adjacent cells.

intracellular space
2–4 nm

adjacent cell
membranes

connexon

a pore
1.5 nm
diameter

sites of interaction). One homophilic binding site is near the N end and has HAV (histidine, alanine and valine) sequences.

Cadherins are attached to actin and cytoplasm inside the cell by a class of linker proteins called catenins. Cadherins are calcium dependent, so changing the extracellular Ca^{2+} concentration will change activity of interactions.

There are four main classes of cadherins:

- E-CAD, which is found in the epithelium and early nervous tissue.

- P-CAD, which is found in epithelium and chicken placenta.
- N-CAD, which is found in nervous tissue and skeletal muscle.
- L-CAM, which is found in liver.

Other cadherins have been identified (e.g. R-CAD in the retina) and proteins related to cadherins have been found in *Drosophila* and desmosomes.

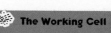

A	Agglutination in blood transfusion			
Donor	**Recipient**			
	O ab	A b	B a	AB o
O ab	–	–	–	–
A b	+	–	+	–
B a	+	+	–	–
A B o	+	+	+	–

Fig. 4.16 Agglutination in blood transfusion illustrated (A) in table form, and (B) diagrammatically. Agglutinogens are denoted by capital letters, and plasma antibodies by small letters.

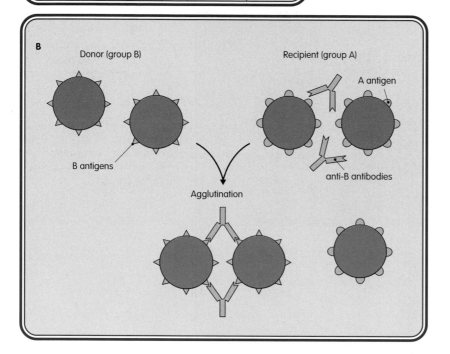

Fig. 4.17 Families of adhesion molecules.

Families of adhesion molecules				
Family	**Members**	**Ca^{2+}/Mg^{2+} dependent**	**Cytoskeletal association**	**Associated cell function**
cadherins	E-CAD, N-CAD, P-CAD	yes	actin filaments	adhesion belts
immunoglobulin (Ig) family	desmosomal CAD	yes	intermediate	desmosomes
selectins (blood and endothelial cells only)	N-CAM, V-CAM, L1	no		none
integrins	P-selectin, E-selectin	yes		none
	LFA-1 (β_2), MAC-1 (β_2)	yes	actin filaments	none

Immunoglobulin (Ig) family

These adhesion molecules are characterized by:

- Antibody fold in each domain.
- β-barrel structure.
- Two β pleated sheets joined by cysteine–cysteine disulphide bonds, which are 60–80 residues apart.
- Loop regions without β structure (variable expressed regions).

There is Ca^{2+}-independent adhesion, and the Ig proteins have homo- and heterophilic binding sites. Heterophilic binding occurs where a protein on one cell acts as a receptor and a different protein on another cell acts as the ligand. Ig members are involved in:

- Adhesion.
- Signalling.
- Axonal growth and fasciculation (fasciculation means that axons grow along other axons by homophilic binding).

N-CAM is an Ig member found in nervous tissue, which can undergo alternative splicing, so expression of exons can vary. It exists in transmembrane, lipid anchored, or secreted forms. Other important Ig family members are listed in Fig. 4.19.

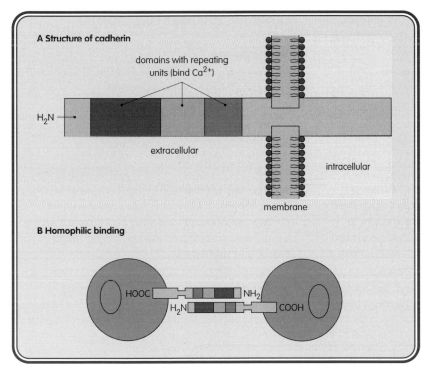

Fig. 4.18 (A) Structure of cadherin. It is composed of five extracellular domains, each 700–750 amino acids in length, and one intracellular domain. The intracellular portion is not present in Tcad (T, truncated). (B) Cadherin exhibits homophilic binding in which the molecule acts as both ligand and receptor.

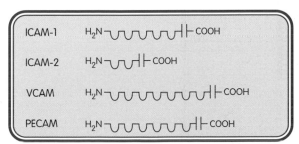

Fig. 4.19 Ig family members. ICAM, intracellular adhesion molecule; VCAM, vascular adhesion molecule; PECAM, platelet endothelial cell adhesion molecule.

Do not be confused by the use of old nomenclature by books or tutors referring to the selectins—P-selectin is also called GMP-140 and E-selectin is also called E-LAM.

Selectins

Selectins are Ca^{2+} independent and undergo heterophilic binding to carbohydrate ligands (Fig. 4.20). P-selectin and E-selectin are cell–cell adhesion molecules expressed by endothelial cells during inflammatory responses, expression being induced by local chemical mediators:

- E-Selectin is activated by tumour necrosis factor (TNF), interleukin-1 (IL-1), and endotoxin.
- P-selectin is activated by histamine, thrombin, platelet activating factor, and phorbol esters.

The lectin domain recognizes specific oligosaccharides on the surface of neutrophils, the oligosaccharides Lewis X and sialyated Lewis X are recognised by P-selectin and E-selectin respectively. Neutrophils thus stick to the endothelial lining of blood vessels via these weak affinity interactions until integrins are activated. L-selectin is constitutive on the surface of polymorphonuclear neutrophils, monocytes, and lymphocytes. Selectins are important in the homing of these cells to lymph nodes and subendothelial capillaries.

Integrins

Integrins are the major receptors for binding to the ECM, and also contribute to some cell–cell interactions. The structure is a heteroduplex of α and β glycoproteins (Fig. 4.21) with a similar structure to transmembrane proteoglycans. There are 14 known α chains and eight known β glycoproteins, each β chain forming an integrin subfamily. Each β has 2–4 α subunits attached (e.g. $\alpha4\beta1$ is a $\beta1$ chain with four α chains attached). The integrins differ from other receptors in that they bind their ligand with low affinity, and are present at high concentration. Interactions are heterophilic and Ca^{2+} dependent (Fig. 4.22). $\beta2$ and $\beta1$ are important integrins.

β2 integrins

These are leucocyte specific. $\beta2\alpha L$ is also called LFA1 (leucocyte function associated). It mediates direct cell–cell interactions by binding ICAM-1 and ICAM-2. MAC1 is also a $\beta2$ integrin and binds ICAM-1. Surface antigen ('cluster of differentiation') nomenclature is also used (e.g. CD18 is $\beta2$).

β1 integrins

These are found on most cells. Several are called VLAs (very late acting) as they are expressed late in lymphocyte activation (e.g. VLA4, which binds VCAM).

Integrins binding

Integrins usually bind actin-based cytoskeleton inside the cell. Outside the cell, integrins can bind:

- ECM (e.g. fibronectin).
- Cell surface molecules (e.g. ICAM-1).
- Soluble molecules (e.g. fibrinogen).

Integrins have recognition sites for ligands (e.g. Ig-like domains bind ICAMs and the tripeptide RGD (arginine, glycine, aspartic acid) which is a sequence commonly expressed in fibronectin and other ECM proteins). Cells can vary their binding properties by varying integrin affinities and specificities.

Integrins take part in signal transduction in cells (e.g. clustering of $\beta1\alpha5$ by fibronectin causes cytoplasmic alkalization).

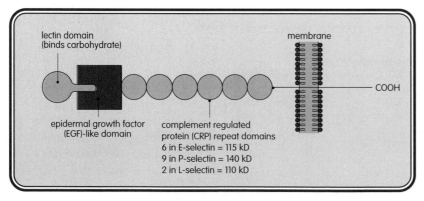

Fig. 4.20 Structure of a selectin molecule.

lectin domain (binds carbohydrate)

membrane

COOH

epidermal growth factor (EGF)-like domain

complement regulated protein (CRP) repeat domains
6 in E-selectin = 115 kD
9 in P-selectin = 140 kD
2 in L-selectin = 110 kD

Basement membrane

Basement membrane is a sheet of ECM underlying epithelial and endothelial cells and surrounds adipocytes, Schwann cells, and muscle cells. It acts to isolate these cells from the mesenchyme or connective tissue. It is also called the basal lamina and is composed of type IV collagen, heparan sulphate, proteoglycans, entactin, and laminin. Functions of basement membrane are:

- Cell adhesion.
- To act as a porous filter in the kidney's glomeruli.
- To inhibit the spread of neoplasia.

- To regulate cell migration.
- Growth and wound healing.
- Differentiation.

Extra Cellular Matrix

ECM is a hydrated polysaccharide gel containing a meshwork of glycoproteins. It is composed of:

- Proteoglycans—which form a gel.
- Structural proteins—collagen, elastin.
- Fibrous adhesive proteins—laminin, fibronectin, tenascin.

Fig. 4.21 Structure of integrin.

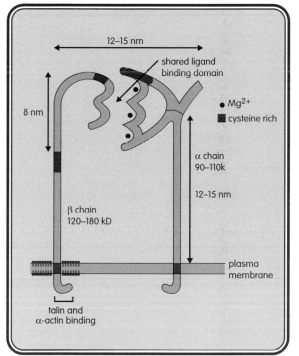

Fig. 4.22 Integrins and transmembrane proteoglycans.

	Integrins and transmembrane proteoglycans				
Family	**Members**	**Ca²⁺/Mg²⁺ dependent**	**Cytoskeletal association**	**Associated cell function**	
integrins	many	yes	actin filaments	focal	
transmembrane proteoglycans	$\alpha_6\beta_4$	yes	intermediate	hemidesmosomes	
	syndecans	no	actin	none	

63

ECM components are secreted by local fibroblasts in most tissues, but chondroblasts and osteoblasts are also involved in cartilage. ECM influences cell division, development, differentiation, migration, metabolism, and shape. Connective tissues rely on the properties of the local ECM, which is:

- Calcified in bone and teeth.
- Ropelike in tendon.
- Transparent, to see through, in the cornea.

Proteoglycans

These form the hydrated polysaccharide gel that acts as a ground substance and allows diffusion of substances such as nutrients and hormones from the blood to the tissue and vice versa. Glycosaminoglycans (GAGs) are unbranched polysaccharide chains of repeating disaccharide units (Fig. 4.23). Proteoglycans are formed in the Golgi apparatus where:

- The core protein is linked via a serine to a tetrasaccharide.
- Glycosyl transferases add sugar residues.
- Ordered sulphation and epimerization reactions occur.

The main types of GAGs are:

- Hyaluronic acid—found as a lubricant in synovial fluid (up to 8×10^6 D).
- Chondroitin sulphate—in cartilage.
- Dermatan sulphate.
- Heparin sulphate—in blood clotting.
- Heparin.
- Keratin sulphate—in skin.

Chondroitin sulphate, dermatan sulphate, and heparin sulphate are all between 500 and 50000 D.

GAGs are very hydrophilic, and have an extended coil structure, which takes up extensive space. GAGs have a negative charge and attract cations; thus Na^+, which is osmotically active, is attracted, so water is sucked into the matrix giving turgor pressure able to withstand forces of many hundreds of times atmospheric pressure.

Proteoglycans function to:

- Provide hydrated space.
- Bind secreted signalling molecules.
- Act as sieves to regulate molecular trafficking. Proteoglycans and glycoproteins are compared in Fig. 4.24.

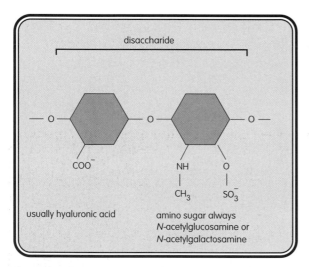

Fig. 4.23 Glycosaminoglycan disaccharide subunit.

Comparison of proteoglycans and glycoproteins	
Proteoglycans	**Glycoproteins**
up to 95% carbohydrate	1–60% carbohydrate by weight
unbranched carbohydrate	branched carbohydrate
80 sugar residues	13 sugar residues
usually no sialic acid	usually 1–10 GAG chains
larger than 3×10^5 D	no larger than 3×10^5 D

Fig. 4.24 Comparison of proteoglycans and glycoproteins.

Collagen

This fibrous protein has great tensile strength, and is resistant to stretching. It comprises 25% of the protein in mammals and is rich in proline (ring structure) and glycine (the smallest amino acid and occurring every third residue so allowing the strands to fit together). Collagen synthesis is carried out in the ER. Synthesis occurs as follows:

- It begins with formation of an amino acid proline α chain.
- Proline and lysine residues are then hydroxylated.
- Finally, interchain hydrogen bonds form a stable triple helix (i.e. procollagen, Fig. 4.25).
- Secretion from the ER causes removal of the propeptides forming collagen. This stage is omitted in type IV collagen.

There are 20 collagen α chains, each encoded by separate genes, but only ten types of collagen. Types I, II, and III are fibrillar collagen and are found in connective tissue (Fig. 4.26).

Fibrils are collagen aggregations of 10–300 nm in diameter and aggregate to form collagen fibres of a few mm in diameter. Organization is tissue specific; for example:

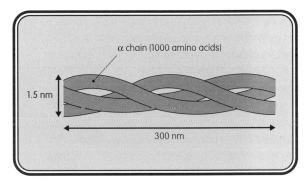

Fig. 4.25 Structure of collagen. Collagen is a right-hand triple helix (superhelix).

- 'Wickerwork' pattern in skin resists multidirectional stress.
- Parallel layers in bone and cornea.

Type IV collagen forms a sheetlike meshwork, and is only found in the basal lamina (Fig. 4.27).

Elastin

Elastin is found in places that need elasticity (e.g. skin, blood vessels, lungs). It is a highly glycosylated, hydrophobic protein (Fig. 4.28) that is rich in the non-hydroxylated forms of proline and glycine. The sheets are organized with the help of a microfibrillar glycoprotein, fibrillin, which is secreted before elastin. Fibrillin deficiency results in Marfan syndrome.

Laminin

Laminin is a complex of three polypeptide chains held together in a 'cross shape' by disulphide bonds.

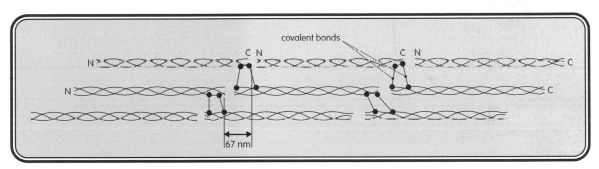

Fig. 4.26 Structure of fibrillar collagen. Collagen molecules are positioned side by side, staggered from adjacent molecules by one-quarter of their length. (Adapted with permission from *Molecular Cell Biology 2e*, by Darnell, Lodish and Baltimore, Scientific American Books, 1990.)

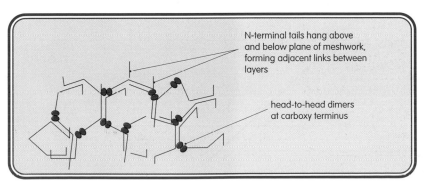

Fig. 4.27 Structure of type IV collagen, which assembles into multilayered sheets. (Adapted with permission from *Molecular Biology of the Cell 3e*, by B. Alberts, D. Bray, J. Lewis, M. Raff, K. Roberts and J.D. Watson, Garland Publishing, 1994.)

Fibronectin

This is an adhesive glycoprotein with binding sites for cells and matrix. It is a dimer of two subunits, which are folded into globular domains. Forms of fibronectin

involved in wound healing and embryogenesis appear to promote cell proliferation and migration.

Tenascin

This protein, which can promote or inhibit cell adhesion and migration, is only produced by embryonic tissue and glial cells.

Role of the fibroblast

Fibroblasts are members of the connective tissue cell family. Members of the connective tissue family are all of common origin and interchangeable under appropriate conditions, other members being chondrocytes, osteocytes, adipocytes, and smooth muscle cells. Connective tissue differentiation is controlled by cytokines, especially hormones and growth factors. Interchangeability allows them to support and repair most tissue types. Fibroblasts:

- Secrete the fibrous proteins of the ECM in most tissues (except in cartilage and bone where they are produced by chondrocytes and osteocytes, respectively).
- Are involved in the organization of ECM, enabling the configuration of ECM into tendons and other structures.

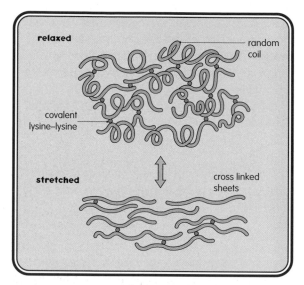

Fig. 4.28 Structure of stretched and relaxed elastin.

- Name the functions of cell interaction and adhesion—list at least four.
- Name and describe the main classes of cell junction.
- Describe the structure of the major cell adhesion molecule families.
- Discuss ECM composition and functions.
- Discuss how fibroblasts control ECM composition.

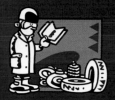
ORGANIZATION OF THE CELL NUCLEUS

Electron microscopy has made it possible to study the ultrastructure of the cell in a way that could never have been possible using light microscopy (see Fig. 1.5).

The nucleus is the largest structure in the eukaryotic cell (Fig. 5.1). It is not a true organelle as it is in constant contact with the cell cytoplasm. It consists of DNA, proteins, and RNA, and plays a vital role in:

- Protein synthesis (see pp. 95–99).
- The passage of genetic information from one generation to the next (see pp. 71–77).

Structures in the nucleus

Nuclear envelope

The nuclear envelope encloses the nucleus. It consists of two layers of membrane, the outer being continuous with the endoplasmic reticulum. Ribosomes are attached to the outer layer of the nuclear envelope as well as to the endoplasmic reticulum. Specific membrane proteins on the inner surface of the envelope form links with structural proteins in the nucleus called lamins.

Nuclear pores

Nuclear pores are found at points of contact between the inner and outer membranes (Fig. 5.2). They are electron-dense structures and consist of eight protein complexes arranged around a central complex. They control the passage of metabolites, macromolecules, and RNA subunits between the nucleus and the cytoplasm.

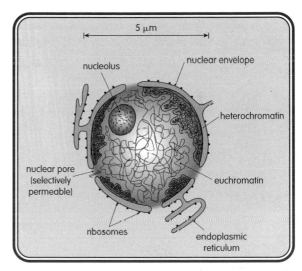

Fig. 5.1 Structure of the nucleus.

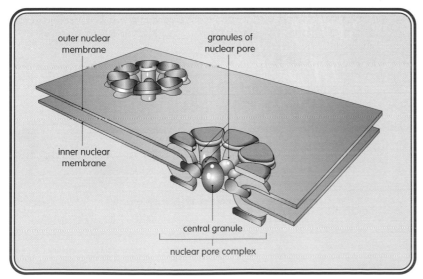

Fig. 5.2 Structure of a nuclear pore.

Chromatin

Chromatin is the collective name for the long strands of DNA and associated proteins called nucleoproteins. Two types of chromatin can be seen when a cell is viewed under an electron microscope:

- Heterochromatin, which is electron dense and is distributed around the periphery of the nucleus and in discrete masses within the nucleus. The DNA is in close association with nucleoproteins and is not active in RNA synthesis. In female cells, small discrete masses of heterochromatin called Barr bodies are seen in the periphery of the nucleus. These represent X chromosomes inactivated by methylation.
- Euchromatin, which is electron lucent and represents DNA that is active in RNA synthesis.

Cells that are not active in protein synthesis tend to have nuclei rich in heterochromatin and no nucleoli. Mature neutrophils are an example with their dense lobulated nuclei (Fig. 5.3).

Nucleoli

Nucleoli are extremely dense structures in the nuclei and are highly active in rRNA synthesis. There may be one, several, or no nucleoli in a cell nucleus. They represent the sites of ribosomal RNA synthesis and assembly.

Nuclear matrix

The nuclear matrix consists of DNA, nucleoproteins, and structural proteins. Nucleoproteins are proteins closely associated with DNA. They are defined as histones and non-histones. Histones are strongly basic globular proteins around which DNA winds in a regular fashion, like beads on a string, to form chromatin (see Fig. 5.16). Chromatin is thought to interact with the protein filaments associated with the inner nuclear envelope called lamins. The lamins are arranged in a lattice and this regular arrangement along with their interactions with chromatin are thought to create a nuclear cytoskeleton.

○ Describe the structure of the cell nucleus in detail and outline the functions of its components.

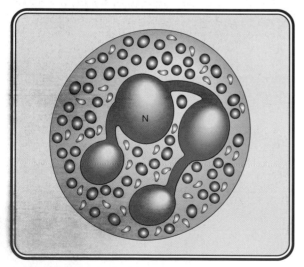

Fig. 5.3 Structure of a mature neutrophil. The nucleus (N) is characteristically multilobed.

CELL CYCLE

Concept of the cell cycle

The cell cycle can be regarded as the life cycle of an individual cell. It can divided into two phases:

- Mitosis (or cell division)—which results in the production of two daughter cells.
- Interphase—the interval between divisions during which the cell undergoes its functions and prepares for mitosis.

The cell cycle can be further subdivided into distinct phases as shown in Fig. 5.4. Restriction points are the boundaries between the phases.

Regulation of the cell cycle

The cell cycle is controlled by gene products, which govern the transition from one phase to another. The intracellular concentrations of these products vary throughout the cell cycle.

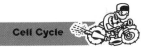

Cyclins

Cyclins control the cell cycle by interacting with cyclin-dependent kinases (CDKs). These in turn are activated and stimulate cell cycle progression by phosphorylation of specific targets in the cell, for example:

- At the beginning of prophase of mitosis, nuclear membrane breakdown is initiated by phosphorylation of lamins, which form part of the nuclear skeleton.
- Chromosome condensation at the beginning of mitosis is initiated by the phosphorylation of H1 histone, a nuclear-associated protein.
- G_1–S transition is initiated by phosphorylation of Rb protein. Unphosphorylated Rb protein forms a complex with the transcription factor E2F. On phosphorylation of Rb, E2F is released and activates transcription of genes required for G_1–S transition.

Human cyclins are designated A to E. Each one accumulates at a different time in the cell cycle (Fig. 5.5).

It is thought that specific CDK inhibitors are always present in the cell. When cyclin levels rise above a threshold the inhibitors can no longer exert their effect, hence the 'spikes' of CDK activity.

Mitosis promoting factor

Mitosis-promoting factor (MPF) is an example of a cyclin–CDK complex. It initiates transition from G_2 into

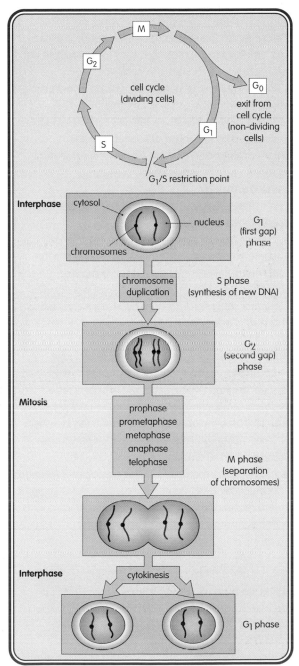

Fig. 5.4 The cell cycle. In G_1 there is cell growth and performance of functions specific to the tissue involved. The length of G_1 varies, depending upon the cell type.

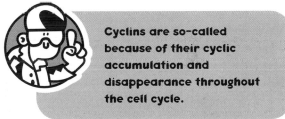

Cyclins are so-called because of their cyclic accumulation and disappearance throughout the cell cycle.

Cyclins and CDKs involved in cell cycle progression		
Cyclin	Kinase	Function
D	CDK4, CDK6	progression past restriction point at G_1/S boundary
E, A	CDK2	initiation of DNA synthesis in early S phase
B	CDK1	transition from G_2 to M

Fig. 5.5 Cyclins and CDKs involved in the cell cycle. Cyclin C does not exist.

mitosis. A small increase in cyclin levels produces a big increase in MPF kinase activity. It is therefore a very powerful factor and can bring about mitosis, even in non-replicating cells. It is under tight control within the cell so that its effects are produced quickly and transiently.

S-phase protein and other factors

S-phase protein controls transition from G_1 into S phase. The cell cycle is influenced by a multitude of other factors including:

- Growth factors.
- Hormones.
- Mitogens (factors that induce mitosis).

The huge variety of factors involved allows cell growth and replication to be finely controlled, responding to changes in the environment. The majority of these factors exert their effect by binding to cell membrane receptors and so producing a signal to the interior of the cell (see Chapter 3).

Growth factors are soluble and diffusible substances that can act locally or over long distances and affect cell growth. They exert their action by binding to specific target receptors on the cell surface, which results in phosphorylation of target proteins within the cell (see Chapter 3).

The cell cycle and cancer

Cancer arises partly as a result of a loss of normal cell cycle control. Normal cells are in equilibrium. There is a balance between proliferation, quiescence, and death. If this balance is disturbed there may be uncontrolled cell growth. Malignant cells may have the ability to grow autonomously (i.e. outside the normal cell cycle controls).

Malignancy occurs as a result of mutation of genomic DNA. Changes in the cell's genomic DNA result in either increased or decreased expression of genes associated with cell cycle control. The most common causes of altered gene expression are:

- Chemical damage (e.g. due to benzene, nitrosamines).
- Radiation (e.g. ultraviolet light).
- Integration of viral DNA into the host genome.
- Inherited defects.

The first three causes listed are 'wear and tear' effects, which mean that the mutations tend to accumulate with age.

Cancer represents clonal expansion of a cell in which there has been sufficient change to the genomic DNA to transform the cell's phenotype from a normal to a malignant cell. Usually in the progression to cancer there is an accumulation of mutations that together cause malignant transformation (see Fig. 6.24).

A number of cancer-causing genes have been identified and their roles discovered.

- Oncogenes are cancer-causing genes whose unregulated expression may lead a cell down the pathway towards malignant transformation.
- Tumour suppressor genes are genes expressed in normal cells and decreased expression can lead to transformation.

Many cancer-causing genes have yet to be found.

p53 is an important tumour suppressor that has been dubbed 'guardian of the genome'. The gene lies on chromosome 17 and codes for a nuclear phosphoprotein of 53 kD. Three major roles of *p53* have been identified:

- Transcription activator—regulating certain genes involved in cell division.
- As a G_1 restriction point for DNA damage—if there has been excess DNA damage (e.g. ultraviolet damage) it inhibits cell division.
- Participation in the initiation of apoptosis.

○ **Describe the concept of the cell cycle and draw a diagrammatic representation of the stages.**
○ **Describe the roles of regulating proteins in the cell cycle and name some examples.**
○ **Explain how the cell cycle plays a role in cancer.**
○ **Give an example of an oncogene and a tumour suppresser gene.**

MITOSIS AND MEIOSIS

Overview of cell division

Cell division is the process by which a cell, including the nucleus, undergoes replication. It is a complex process because, for the daughter cells to be viable, each must contain a complete set of genetic material so that proteins can be manufactured and the new cell can carry out its function. The concept of the cell cycle as a continuous process of growth and replication has been mentioned previously (see Fig. 5.4). Here, mitosis and meiosis, the mechanisms by which genetic material is distributed as cells divide, are discussed:

- Mitosis is the type of cell division that occurs in somatic cells and results in the production of two genetically identical daughter cells.
- Meiosis occurs in gamete formation (e.g. sperm and ova). Each daughter cell contains half the genetic information of the parent cell and crossing-over ensures a reassortment of genetic material between the chromosomes of each homologous pair.

Definitions

Important definitions in meiosis and mitosis include the following:

- Karyotype—this is the chromosome complement of a cell. In a standard karyotype the chromosomes are conventionally arranged in an order depending upon size, shape, and banding patterns.
- Genome—this is the entire genetic complement of a cell.
- Gamete—the reproductive cell formed by meiosis containing half the normal chromosome number.
- Ploidy—this refers to the number of complete sets of chromosomes in a cell. A haploid cell contains a single set of chromosomes (e.g. gametes); a diploid cell contains two copies of each chromosome (e.g. somatic cells); a polyploid cell contains more than two sets of chromosomes (sometimes this occurs normally in plants).

Mitosis

Two identical daughter cells are formed as a result of mitosis.

Mitosis: 2n → 2n

There are four distinct phases in mitosis (Fig. 5.6).

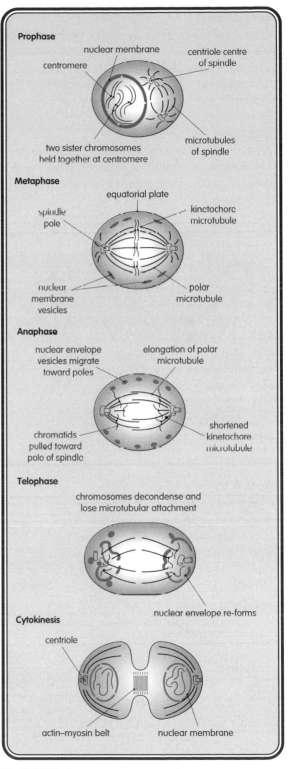

Fig. 5.6 Mitosis.

Prophase

There is condensation of chromosomes and the centrioles duplicate and migrate towards opposite poles of the cell. A spindle of microtubules is formed simultaneously.

Dissolution of the nuclear membrane marks the end of prophase.

Metaphase

The chromosomes become attached to the spindle. The area of attachment is called the kinetochore. The chromosomes become arranged along the spindle, forming the equatorial plate.

Anaphase

Chromatids separate at the centromeres and are pulled to opposite poles by the spindle. The end of anaphase is marked by the clustering of two groups of identical chromatids at opposite poles of the cell.

Telophase

The chromosomes begin to uncoil. The nuclear membrane re-forms and nucleoli reappear. The cytoplasm is divided into two by the process of cytokinesis.

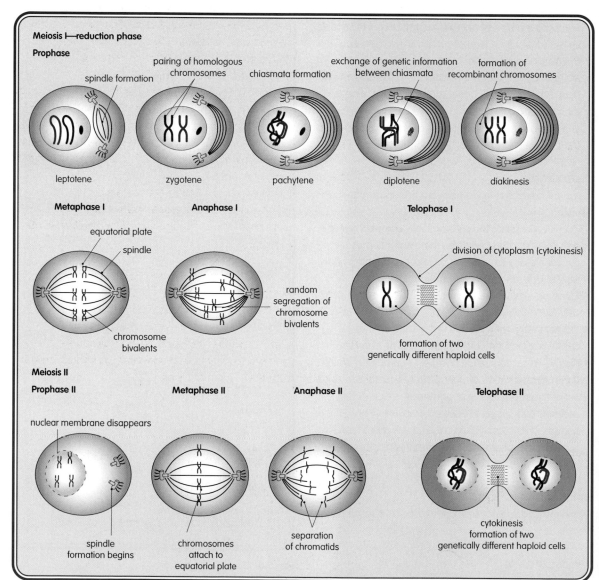

Fig. 5.7 Meiosis—see text for explanation of each phase.

Meiosis

In the first division of meiosis two genetically different haploid cells are formed (Fig. 5.7). In the second division, each haploid cell is duplicated.

Meiosis: $2n \rightarrow n$

Prophase I

There are five stages during which homologous chromosomes come together and exchange segments in homologous recombination:

- Leptotene—spindle forms.
- Zygotene—homologous chromosomes pair, shorten, and thicken, and form bivalents (pairs of homologous chromosomes).
- Pachytene—chiasmata begin to form. These are points at which non-homologous chromatids become associated with each other via base pairing. These become points of 'crossing-over' between the chromatids.
- Diplotene—exchange of genetic material in chiasmata and nucleolar membrane disappears.
- Diakinesis—recombinant chromosomes are formed.

Metaphase I

Chromosomes become attached to a spindle (see mitotic metaphase).

Anaphase I

The chromatids do not separate and whole chromosomes migrate to opposite poles of spindle, hence 'reduction division'.

Telophase I

Two genetically different haploid cells are formed.

Second division

The second division is like mitosis, but a haploid number of chromosomes are involved. The chromatids separate in anaphase II.

Two processes in meiosis are vital in the generation of genetic diversity:

- Chiasmata formation ('crossing-over'), which allows random exchange of genetic material between homologous chromosomes.
- Independent segregation of homologous chromosomes.

During anaphase I, homologous chromosomes segregate independently of each other. Since humans possess 23 pairs of homologous chromosomes, there are 2^{23} possible ways that the chromosomes can segregate to form a haploid set.

In humans, meiosis begins during gametogenesis. In females this occurs in the ovaries. The first ('reduction') meiotic division begins during month 5 of embryonic life, but is arrested at pro-metaphase and is completed just before ovulation. Meiosis II takes place after ovulation. Therefore:

- There are a fixed number of oocytes.
- There is a period of arrest between the start of meiosis I and the completion of meiosis II of 12–45 years.

Oogenesis produces a single oocyte and two polar bodies (Fig. 5.8).

Male spermatogenesis occurs in the seminiferous tubules of the testes. After sexual maturity the spermatogonia continuously multiply by mitosis, subsequently undergoing meiosis to produce unlimited numbers of spermatocytes.

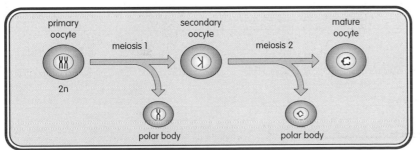

Fig. 5.8 Oogenesis.

Endomitosis

Endomitosis is the process of repeated DNA replication in the absence of nuclear division and cytokinesis. It can generate huge nuclei with up to 16 copies of the DNA. Endomitosis occurs in the formation of megakaryocytes, which are cells in the bone marrow from which anucleate platelets bud off.

- ○ **Define mitosis and meiosis.**
- ○ **Describe the stages involved in mitosis and meiosis and compare the two processes.**
- ○ **Define endomitosis.**

STRUCTURE AND PROPERTIES OF NUCLEIC ACIDS

Structure of nucleic acids

Nucleic acids are linear polymers of nucleotides (Fig. 5.9). There are two types called DNA (deoxyribonucleic acid) and RNA (ribonucleic acid) and they form an integral part of the growth and replication of all living cells.

Nucleotides have three components:
- Base (purine or pyrimidine).
- Pentose sugar.
- Phosphate.

Purines and pyrimidines

These are the two types of bases found in nucleic acids.

They are planar aromatic rings that contain nitrogen. The five bases that occur in nucleic acids are shown in Fig. 5.10.

Purine and pyrimidine biosynthesis

Almost all eukaryotic cells are capable of synthesizing purines and pyrimidines *de novo*. This shows how important they are to cell survival.

Purines are synthesized in an 11-stage pathway with a starting chemical of α-D-ribose-phosphate. The process requires folate (tetrahydrofolate). The initial product is inositol monophosphate (IMP), which is rapidly converted to adenosine monophosphate (AMP) and guanosine monophosphate (GMP). A complex negative feedback control network operates to prevent excessive build-up of AMP and GMP.

Pyrimidine synthesis involves a six-step pathway in which the ribose sugar is incorporated as one of the final steps. The final product is uracil triphosphate (UTP), which is converted to CTP (cytosine triphosphate) by amination of the uracil.

Pentose sugars

These are five-carbon rings (see Fig. 5.9). Deoxyribonucleotides are formed by the reduction of the ribose group of the corresponding ribonucleotide.

Nucleosides and nucleotides

Nucleic acid production involves nucleoside triphosphates. During synthesis a series of nucleic acid condensation reactions occur between phosphate and sugar groups to produce very strong covalent bonds called phosphodiester bonds. Long, unbranching chains form with linkages between C3 and C5 of each sugar, hence the notation 5'→3' or 3'→5' to describe the

Fig. 5.9 Structure of a nucleotide. Deoxyribose has an -H group on ^{2}C, while ribose has an -OH group on ^{2}C.

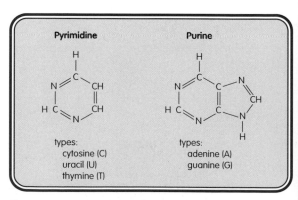

Fig. 5.10 Structure of pyrimide and purine bases.

orientation of nucleotides in a nucleic acid chain. Each sugar is separated from the next by a phosphate group to form a strong and rigid sugar–phosphate backbone from which the bases project (Fig. 5.11).

DNA double helix

The structure of DNA was discovered by Watson and Crick in 1953. They showed that DNA in eukaryotic cells consists of two intertwined polynucleotide strands held together by base pairing to form a double helix. Adenine and thymine bases, and guanine and cytosine pair via non-covalent hydrogen bonds (Fig. 5.12). Base pairing results in two complementary polynucleotides, which run antiparallel to each other (i.e. one runs 5' to 3', the other runs 3' to 5'; Fig. 5.11).

**Remember this phrase!
DNA is a double helix consisting of two complementary antiparallel polynucleotide strands.**

Nucleotides and nucleosides. A nucleotide can also be called a 'nucleoside monophosphate'. Nucleosides can be multiplied, phosphorylated, and the breakdown of phosphate bonds drives many cellular reactions including DNA synthesis.

5' and 3' notation will be important when transcription and translation are discussed later.

DNA as an information carrier

DNA is found predominantly in the nucleus. It acts as a template during transcription and is also the vehicle of inheritance (i.e. it is passed from one generation to the next.

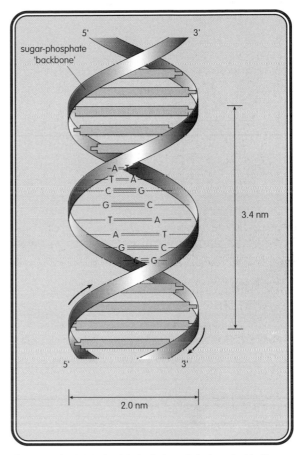

Fig. 5.11 The DNA double helix is a right-handed helix with a common axis for both strands. There are ten base pairs per turn. (A, adenine; C, cytosine; G, guanine; T, thymine.)

Comparison of DNA and RNA		
Feature	**DNA**	**RNA**
sugar	deoxyribose	ribose
base pairing	A–T/G–C	A–U/G–C
structure	double helix	single stranded structures

Fig. 5.12 Comparison of DNA and RNA. (A, adenine; C, cytosine; G, guanine; T, thymine.)

RNA molecules

RNA is synthesized predominantly in the nucleus and moves out into the cytoplasm to carry out its function. In eukaryotic cells, all RNA is produced from DNA by transcription.

Messenger RNA

Messenger RNA (mRNA) carries genetic information from the nucleus into the cytoplasm. It is derived by splicing from the initial RNA transcript and forms the template upon which polypeptides are manufactured during translation. It is a single stranded molecule without any intramolecular hydrogen bonds (Fig. 5.13).

Transfer RNA

Transfer RNA (tRNA):

- Carries specific amino acids to the site of protein synthesis.
- Has two active sites, which allow it to carry out its functions.
- Is a linear molecule with an average of 76 nucleotides.
- Exhibits extensive intramolecular base pairing, which gives it a characteristic 'clover-leaf'-shaped secondary structure.

Up to 20% of the bases undergo post-translational modification. Their precise function is not known, but they may be involved in tRNA–protein interactions or stabilizing the tRNA molecule. Fig. 5.14 shows the arrangement of the secondary structure of tRNA.

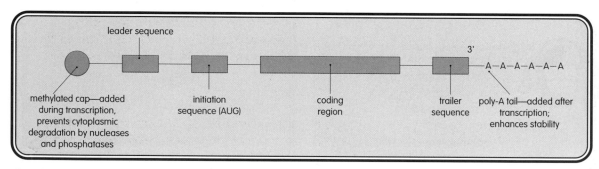

Fig. 5.13 Structure of eukaryotic mRNA. (A, adenine; G, guanine; U, uracil)

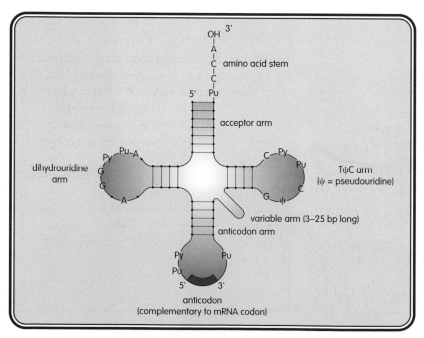

Fig. 5.14 Secondary structure of tRNA. It consists of five arms. The active sites are on the acceptor arm, where the 3' terminal CCA group can accept a specific amino acid, and the anticodon is on the anticodon arm, which recognizes the corresponding mRNA codon. Specific base pairing within the five arms help to maintain the secondary structure. (A, adenine; C, cytosine; Cφ pseudouridine; G, guanine; Pu, purine; Py, pyrimidine; U, uridine.)

Ribosomal RNA

Ribosomal RNA (rRNA) is associated with ribosomes. In a eukaryotic cell each ribosome consists of two unequal subunits, made up of proteins and RNA, called the S (small) and L (large) subunits (Fig. 5.15). The RNA molecules undergo extensive intramolecular base pairing, which is important in determining the ribosomal structure. Ribosomes are capable of self-assembly under physiological conditions with the correct complement of components.

Heteronuclear RNA

Heteronuclear RNA (hnRNA) is the primary transcript produced by eukaryotic cells. Functional RNA is produced by a process called 'splicing'—see p. 90.

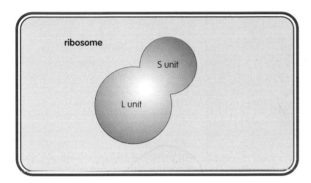

Fig. 5.15 Structure of a ribosome. In rat cytoplasmic ribosome, the units are as follows: S unit 40 S–33 polypeptides and 18 S RNA; L unit 60 S–49 polypeptides and three rRNAs of 2.8 S, 5.8 S, and 5 S. (S = Svedberg unit of sedimentation fraction.)

- ° **Nucleic acid structure— define bases, purines, pyrimidines, nucleosides, and nucleotides.**
- ° **Explain how nucleotides are arranged in the DNA double helix.**
- ° **Draw simple diagrams to show the structure of mRNA and tRNA molecules.**
- ° **Name the components of eukaryotic rRNA.**

DNA PACKAGING AND REPAIR

DNA packaging in the nucleus
Concepts

In the nucleus of a normal human cell, there are 46 chromosomes each containing 48–240 million bases of DNA. According to Watson and Crick's DNA double helix model, each chromosome would have a contour length of 1.6–8.2 cm (i.e. the total length of the DNA would be about 3 m), but the average nucleus has a diameter of approximately 5 μm! An extremely high degree of organization is needed to fit this amount of DNA into a nucleus in a way that makes transcription and DNA replication possible. DNA packaging can be described on three levels.

Nucleosomes

Level one of DNA organization is achieved by nucleosome formation in which the DNA wraps itself around protein complexes called nucleosome core particles.

Chromatin

Chromatin is the DNA, RNA, and protein complex formed in the eukaryotic nucleus. H1 histones bind to DNA as it winds around the core particle and also bind to other H1s to allow the DNA to achieve its second level of organization (Fig. 5.16).

Histones

Histones are positively charged proteins and can therefore make ionic bonds with the negative phosphate groups in nucleic acids. The $(H2A)_2 (H2B)_2 (H3)_2 (H4)_2$ octamer is capable of self-assembly in the correct conditions and in the presence of both:

- Nucleoplasmin, an acidic protein that allows the histones and DNA to come together in a controlled way.
- DNA topoisomerase I, a nicking–closing enzyme that helps in DNA supercoiling.

The histone proteins are well conserved through species, which shows that their structure and function are vital to life.

Loop formation

The third level of organization is loop formation in which the DNA forms loops radiating from a central scaffold of non-histone proteins. It is thought that the loops form transcriptional units.

Chromosomes

During cell division, chromatin condenses to form rod-shaped organelles called chromosomes, which stain with biological dyes such as Giemsa. Each chromosome corresponds to a single strand of chromatin. They are most densely packed at metaphase and after staining can be easily viewed under a light microscope.

Each chromosome is composed of two identical strands of DNA called sister chromatids. Chromatids are connected at a central region called the centromere, above and below which chromatin strands loop across between chromatids to hold them together (Fig. 5.17).

The kinetochore is an organelle located at the centromere region. It acts as a microtubule organizing centre (MTOC) and facilitates spindle formation by polymerization of tubulin dimers to form microtubules during the early stages of mitosis (see Chapter 4).

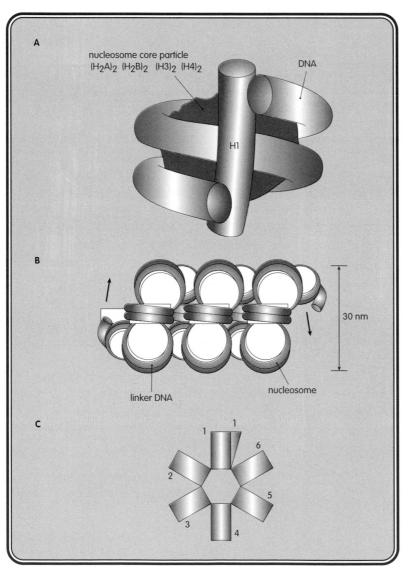

Fig. 5.16 Chromatin fibre organization. (A) The nucleosome core particle is composed of pairs of histones—$(H2A)_2$ $(H2B)_2$ $(H3)_2$ $(H4)_2$. A fifth histone, H1, is also associated with the nucleosome. 166 base pairs of DNA wind around each nucleosome. Linker DNA runs between one nucleosome and the next. It consists of 8–114 base pairs. (B) Chromatin consists of nucleosomes bound together through their H1 proteins (not shown in this part of the figure). (C) Bound nucleosomes form a solenoid, with six nucleosomes per turn. (Adapted with permission from *Molecular Biology of the Cell 3e* , by B. Alberts, D. Bray, J. Lewis, M. Raff, K Roberts and J.D. Watson, Garland Publishing, 1994.)

DNA damage

Agents that cause DNA damage include:

- Ionizing radiation.
- Ultraviolet light, which promotes chemical cross-linking between two adjacent thymine residues on a DNA strand, resulting in the formation of a pyrimidine dimer. These distort the DNA double helix in the region of the dimer.
- Chemical mutagens, which can be of three types: base analogues (e.g. 5-bromouracil)—become incorporated into the DNA and cause misreading; chemical modifiers (e.g. hydroxylamine)—react with bases to form derivatives that cause misreading; Intercalators (e.g. some antibiotics)—slip between adjacent bases and inhibit RNA transcription.
- Parts of (or entire) viral genomes, which can become incorporated into eukaryotic chromatin. This can disrupt coding regions or promoting regions or can affect levels of expression of existing genes.

DNA can also change spontaneously under normal physiological conditions. For example, adenine and cytosine can undergo spontaneous deamination to produce hypoxanthine and uracil residues.

A mutation is a change in the base sequence of DNA:

- If this is in a coding region and there is a change in the number of bases, this may result in a frameshift error in which the sequence of triplets of bases coding for each amino acid is disrupted. This usually results in a truncated protein product.
- An altered base may result in a misreading error, which can result in an altered protein product.
- The mutation may disrupt a regulatory region and affect the level of expression of a particular gene.

DNA repair

Any DNA damage must be corrected if DNA is to maintain its integrity. Fig. 5.18 shows the three mechanisms by which mammalian cells can replace abnormal regions of DNA.

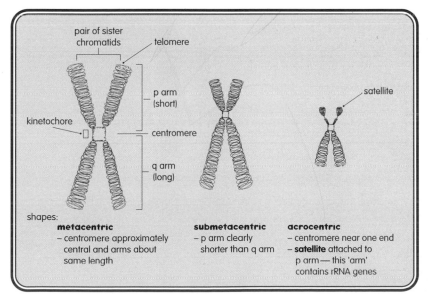

Fig. 5.17 Anatomy of a chromosome, to show the three shapes: metacentric, submetacentric and acrocentric.

79

Name	Problem	Repair mechanism	Disease associated with defect in mechanism
mismatch repair	copy errors causing small unpaired loops in newly synthesized DNA	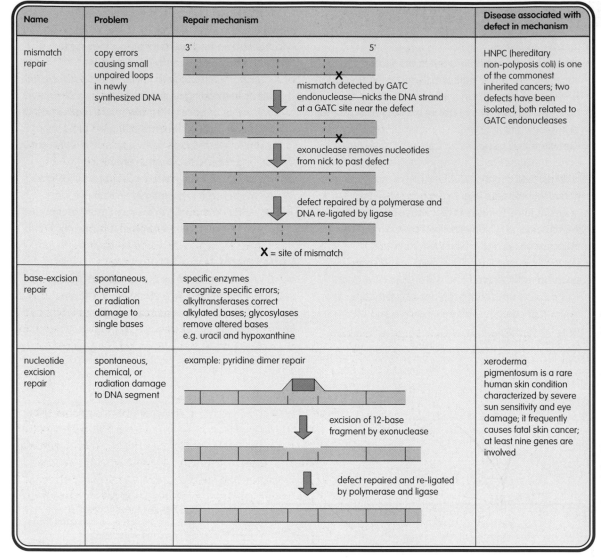	HNPC (hereditary non-polyposis coli) is one of the commonest inherited cancers; two defects have been isolated, both related to GATC endonucleases
base-excision repair	spontaneous, chemical or radiation damage to single bases	specific enzymes recognize specific errors; alkyltransferases correct alkylated bases; glycosylases remove altered bases e.g. uracil and hypoxanthine	
nucleotide excision repair	spontaneous, chemical, or radiation damage to DNA segment	example: pyridine dimer repair excision of 12-base fragment by exonuclease defect repaired and re-ligated by polymerase and ligase	xeroderma pigmentosum is a rare human skin condition characterized by severe sun sensitivity and eye damage; it frequently causes fatal skin cancer; at least nine genes are involved

Fig. 5.18 Mammalian DNA defect repair mechanisms. GATC (guanine, adenine, thymine and cytosine) exonuclease recognizes and binds to a GATC base sequence near to the DNA defect and nicks the DNA at this site.

- Describe how DNA is packaged in the nucleus.
- List four agents that cause DNA damage and give examples of each.
- Discuss the three DNA repair mechanisms and diseases associated with faulty repair mechanisms.

DNA REPLICATION

DNA replication is a complex process that requires about 30 proteins in prokaryotes (and many more proteins in eukaryotes). The complexity of the process is vital to ensure that DNA is copied with high fidelity. A DNA strand can act as a template to direct synthesis of a complementary strand. This process is called semi-conservative replication.

Initiation of replication

In order for a piece of double stranded DNA (dsDNA) to replicate itself according to the semi-conservative theory, the following events must take place :

- An origin of replication must be identified.
- dsDNA must unwind to provide a single stranded DNA (ssDNA) template.
- Initiation of DNA synthesis (which involves synthesis of an RNA primer).

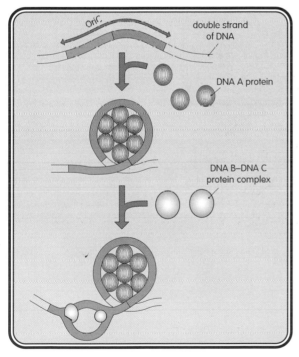

Fig. 5.19 Formation of pre-priming complex for prokaryotic DNA replication. DNA A is a protein that recognizes and binds to nine-base-pair segments of OriC. The process is facilitated by Hu protein. The DNA A–DNA complex becomes negatively supercoiled. The DNA A–DNA complex guides the binding of DNA B–DNA C complex onto the adjacent region of OriC. DNA B has helicase activity and unwinds the DNA in the pre-priming complex. (Adapted with permission from *Biochemistry* by Dr D.Voet and Dr J.C. Voet, John Wiley & Sons, 1990.)

Prokaryotic initiation

Escherichia coli is often used as a model for prokaryotic DNA replication as it has a single chromosome and it divides approximately every 20 minutes at 37°C. It has a single origin of replication called OriC, which is a 245-base-pair segment. Sequence-specific protein binding around the origin causes the DNA to denature (strands dissociate) and unwind. This produces a pre-priming complex, which facilitates further unwinding and entry of a primase and RNA polymerase, resulting in the synthesis of an RNA primer (Fig. 5.19).

Eukaryotic initiation

Eukaryotic DNA replication involves multiple origins. Initiation at the origins is separated spatially and temporally. Clusters of up to 100 origins undergo initiation at the same time. The coordinating trigger is unknown, but there is thought to be an intrinsic factor in the DNA. The genome is replicated once only and it is thought that the chromatin is marked after replication to prevent it being replicated a second time, possibly by DNA methylation (Fig. 5.20).

DNA polymerases

DNA replication is achieved by enzymes called DNA-dependent polymerases. They are DNA dependent because they use ssDNA as a template upon which to form a complementary strand of DNA. They couple nucleoside triphosphates onto a growing DNA strand by addition of a phosphate group onto the free 3'-OH group at the end of the growing DNA strand. The reaction is driven by the elimination of a pyrophosphate (PP_i) and its subsequent hydrolysis. The overall reaction is:

$$(DNA)_n + dNTP \rightarrow (DNA)_{n+1} + PP_i$$

Prokaryotic polymerases

E. coli polymerases are described in Fig. 5.21. The thermophilic bacterium *Thermus aquaticus* has a heat-stable DNA polymerase, which has been very important in the development of molecular genetics. The isolated enzyme, *Taq* polymerase, is used in the polymerase chain reaction, which is described in Chapter 6 (p. 134).

Eukaryotic polymerases

There are four types of polymerase in animal cells, designated α, β, γ, and δ, which have been classified by their response to different inhibitors (Fig. 5.22).

81

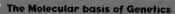

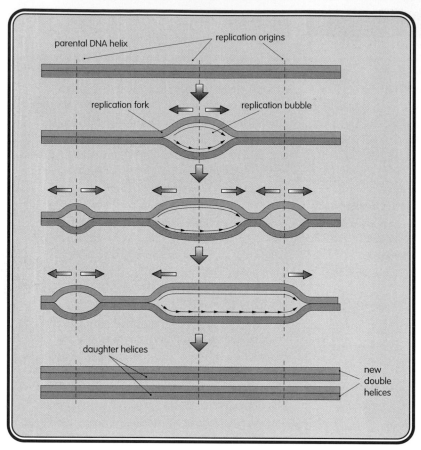

Fig. 5.20 Eukaryotic DNA replication. There are multiple origins of replication, but replication is initiated at specific points at specific times to ensure that the entire genome is replicated once, and once only. (Adapted from *Medical Genetics* by Jorde, Mosby Year Book, 1997.)

Polymerases in *Escherichia coli* (prokaryote)		
	Pol I	**Pol III**
notes	first polymerase to be discovered by Kornberg in 1957	discovered when a mutant strain of *E. coli* with very low Pol I activity was shown to have a normal rate of reproduction
structure	single polypeptide with 928 residues, 109 kD mass; forms one large ('Klenow') fragment and one small fragment	three subunits with total 140 kD; subunits—a, e, q
functions	polymerase (Klenow fragment) 3'–5' exonuclease (Klenow) 5'–3' exonuclease (small fragment)	polymerase (a subunit), 3'–5' exonuclease (e subunit) 5'–3' exonuclease
associated proteins	nil	at least seven other proteins associate to form a complex called the Pol III holoenzyme
processivity (the number of consecutive reactions the enzyme is capable of performing)	at least 20 consecutive polymerization steps can occur before Pol I becomes dissociated from the DNA	in the holoenzyme the extra subunits interact with DNA and other proteins to clamp the polymerase onto the DNA, creating very high processivity (> 5000 residues); Pol III alone has a processivity of 10–15 residues
main biological function	proofreading and error correction	DNA replication

Fig. 5.21 Prokaryotic polymerases. *E.coli* also has a Pol II. Its main physiological function is unknown.

Eukaryotic polymerases				
	α	β	γ	δ
notes	multi-subunit protein; activity varies with rate of cell proliferation	activity does not affect rate of cell growth	chloroplasts contain similar enzymes	
mass (kD)	120–220	30–50	150–300	140–160
inhibitors				
aphidicolin dideoxy	yes	no	no	yes
dideioxol NTPs	weak	strong	strong	weak
arabinosyl NTPs	strong	weak	weak	strong
NEM	strong	weak	strong	strong
functions	polymerase, primase, NO exonuclease	polymerase, exonuclease	polymerase	polymerase 3'–5' exonuclease
location	nucleus	nucleus	mitochondrion	nucleus
processivity	moderate (approximately 100 nucleotides)	?	unlimited	?
biological function	replication of 'lag strand' DNA (see pp. 84–85).	DNA repair	replication of mitochondrial DNA	'lead strand' replication

Fig. 5.22 Eukaryotic polymerases. (NEM, *N*-ethyl-maleimide) . NTP, nucleoside triphosphate

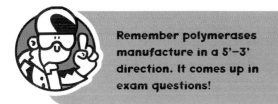

Remember polymerases manufacture in a 5'–3' direction. It comes up in exam questions!

Polymerization process

DNA-dependent polymerases can manufacture DNA only in a 5'–3' direction, which means that the polymerase complex moves along its template strand 3'–5'. The semi-discontinuous theory explains how both strands can be replicated simultaneously (Fig. 5.23). DNA complementary to the lead strand extends in a 5'–3' direction and is synthesized continuously. DNA synthesis on the lag strand is also 5'–3', but in fragments of 1–2 kilobases called Okasaki fragments .

Telomerases are enzymes that replace the 5' end of the lag strand following DNA replication. This is important in the maintenance of viable cells through the generations as the lag strand would otherwise become progressively shorter until DNA replication was no longer possible. Telomerases have been implicated in tumour growth as their presence may immortalize cell lines so that a limitless number of cells can be produced from a single progenitor.

Proofreading and error correction

In both prokaryotes and eukaryotes two processes maintain the fidelity of DNA replication.

- The first is specific base pairing during DNA replication, which is dependent upon the correct complement of dNTPs.
- The second is a 'proofreading process', which in prokaryotes is performed by the polymerase complex.

Fig. 5.21 shows that both Pol I and Pol III have 3'–5' exonucleases. The 3'–5' exonuclease Pol I is activated by an unpaired nucleotide at the 3' end of a newly synthesized DNA strand. The polymerase is inhibited until the erroneous nucleotide is excised; then the polymerase can recommence its function Pol I can correct its mistakes as it goes along but it also

83

removes 10% of correctly paired bases. The 3'–5' exonuclease occurs on Pol I's Klenow fragment, along with the polymerase.

Pol I also has a 5'–3' exonuclease in its small fragment. It can bind to dsDNA at single strand nicks and remove single or several nucleotides. It also removes the RNA primers at the 5' ends of Okasaki fragments and replaces them with DNA in a process called nick translation. This process increases the fidelity of DNA replication as it decreases the chance of non-specific base pairing (see Fig 5.23).

Mammalian polymerases are not capable of proof-reading. This process is done by endonucleases such

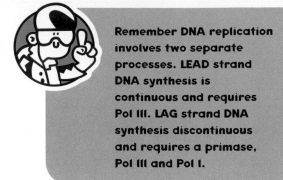

Remember DNA replication involves two separate processes. LEAD strand DNA synthesis is continuous and requires Pol III. LAG strand DNA synthesis discontinuous and requires a primase, Pol III and Pol I.

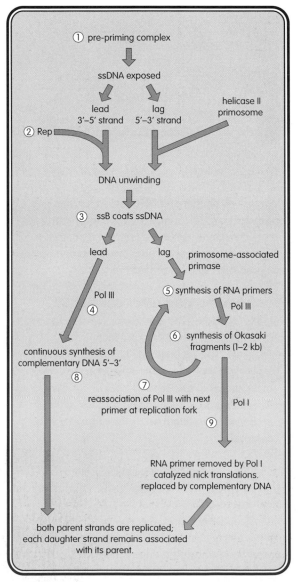

Fig. 5.23 Prokaryotic polymerization process in *E. coli*. (1) DNA is supercoiled around DNA A. DNA B and DNA C facilitate ssDNA exposure. (2) REP protein binds to the lead strand. Helicase II and primosome bind to the lag strand. These produce further unwinding of the DNA. (3) Single strand binding protein (ssB) coats the ssDNA and prevents re-association. (4) The Pol III holoenzyme replicates DNA in *E. coli*. There is continuous synthesis of the DNA complementary to the lead strand (5'–3'). (5) Lag strand synthesis is initiated by synthesis of an RNA primer by a primase. (6) The lag strand is replicated in fragments ('Okasaki fragments'), each of which has a 5' RNA primer. (7) The Pol III dissociates from the newly synthesized Okasaki fragment and reassociates with the next RNA primer at the replication fork. (8) DNA synthesis of both the lead and lag strands occurs on the same multiprotein called a replisome. Therefore the lag strand has to loop around on itself to become associated with the replisome. (See Fig. 5.24.)

as GATC endonuclease and the process is called mismatch repair (see Fig. 5.18).

The rate of copying error after double monitoring is 1 in 10^8–10^{10} base pairs. A human with 10^{14} nucleated cells can accumulate one mutation per 10^6 base pairs within a lifetime.

Consider the DNA replication process in three stages: initiation, elongation and termination.

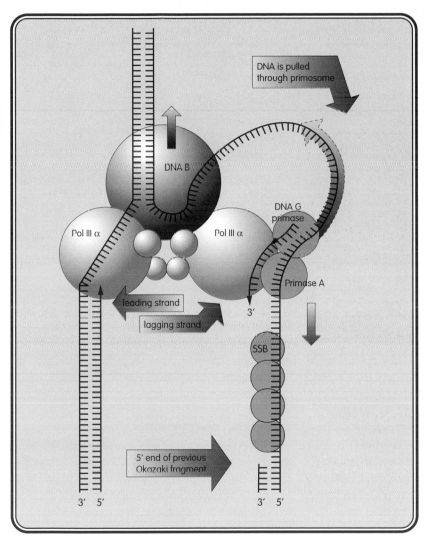

Fig. 5.24 Replication of DNA in *E. coli*. (Adapted with permission from *Genes V*, by B. Lewin, Oxford University Press. 1994.)

- Describe the mechanism involved in initiation of replication. Compare prokaryotes and eukaryotes.
- Give examples of prokaryotic and eukaryotic DNA polymerases. Relate their structure to their function.
- Describe the polymerization process in terms of stages and factors involved.
- What is meant by proofreading and error correction?

Comparison of prokaryotic and eukarytic DNA replication		
	E. coli (prokaryote)	mammalian (eukaryote)
site	cytoplasm	nucleus (and mitochondrion)
no. of proteins involved	30	100s
DNA polymerase	Pol I—fidelity and repair Pol II—DNA synthesis	four enzymes identified, α polymerase is the principal nuclear polymerase.
initiation	single origin of replication (OriC)	multiple origins of replication (spatially and temporally separated during DNA replication)
other materials required	RNA primers, ddNTPs	RNA primers, ddNTPS
mode of replication	semi-conservative	semi-conservative
rate of replication	10^3 nucleotides/sec	10^2 nucleotides/sec
direction of synthesis	5' to 3'. Continuous synthesis of LEAD strand. DISCONTINUOUS synthesis of LAG strand.	5' to 3'. CONTINUOUS synthesis of LEAD strand from each origin. DISCONTINUOUS synthesis of LAG strand
post-replication	RNA primers removed from lag strand by Pol I 5'–3' exonuclease.	RNA primers removed by 5'–3' exonuclease (NOT associated with α polymerase)
timing of replication	continuous DNA synthesis between cell divisions	DNA synthesis and cell division separated by G1 and G2 (gap) phases

Fig. 5.25 Prokaryotic and eukaryotic DNA replication.

TRANSCRIPTION OF DNA

Overview

Transcription

Transcription is the process by which RNA is synthesized under the direction of a DNA template. The process is catalysed by DNA-dependent RNA polymerases, which unwind dsDNA to expose unpaired bases upon which DNA–RNA hybrids form. RNA is synthesized 5'–3'. The DNA template displays polarity in that only one strand can act as a template (template strand). The other strand is called the coding strand as it has the same base composition as the RNA except that thymines (Ts) are substituted for uracils (Us).

Translation

Translation is the mRNA-directed biosynthesis of polypeptides. It is a complex process that involves several hundred macromolecules.

Prokaryotic transcription

Transcription occurs in three phases:

- Initiation.
- Elongation.
- Termination.

E. coli RNA polymerase (RNAP)

E. coli RNA polymerase (RNAP) is a large holoenzyme that contains two Zn^{2+} ions, which the enzyme needs for its catalytic activity. It has a core subunit composition of $\alpha_2\beta\beta'$, which associates with another subunit s, to form the initiation complex, $\alpha_2\beta\beta's$. It binds to the TATAAT box (sequences of bases TATAAT) in the promoter region. The complex also binds to the DNA template and β binds the nucleotides.

Initiation

Subunit s binds to the promoter region. This induces a conformational change in RNAP, which allows nucleotides to associate with the β subunit. This is followed by chemical initiation, which involves coupling of two nucleotide triphosphates. The first is almost always a purine, usually adenine:

$$pppA + pppN \rightarrow pppApN + PP_i$$
pppA = adenosine triphosphate
pppN = nucleoside triphosphate

s factor dissociates.

Elongation
The RNA molecule is synthesized 5'–3'. The DNA template is gradually unwound by RNAP pushing the DNA's coils ahead of it, creating positive superhelicity ahead of the complex and corresponding unwinding behind it. Only about 17 bases are exposed at a time. The RNA quickly leaves the DNA template and the DNA re-forms its double helix.

The overall equation for the polymerization process is:

$$(RNA)_n + XTP \rightarrow (RNA)_{n+1} + PP_i \rightarrow 2P_i$$
XTP = nucleoside triphosphate

Hydrolysis of pyrophosphate drives the reaction to completion (Fig. 5.26)

Termination
The DNA template codes for a termination signal in the RNA transcript. At the end of the RNA transcript there is a guanine-rich region followed by an adenine/thymine-rich region. These two regions can form base pairs to produce a stable hairpin structure. At the very end of

- In prokaryotic cells both transcription and translation take place in the cytoplasm.
- In eukaryotic cells, transcription takes place in the nucleus and translation occurs in the cytoplasm. The two processes are separate and DNA never comes into contact with ribosomes.

the transcript is an oligo(uracil) tail, which forms weak base pairs with the DNA transcript and encourages the RNA to leave the DNA.

The Rho (ρ) factor is an enzyme that encourages termination with or without a hairpin. It has a recognition sequence in the RNA, which the ρ factor binds to and then moves up the RNA 5'–3' until it encounters RNA polymerase. It unwinds the DNA–RNA complex and releases the RNA.

Prokaryotic post-transcriptional modification
In prokaryotes there is very little or no post-transcriptional modification of mRNA and translation occurs as the RNA transcript is produced. rRNA and tRNA are synthesized as a continuous strand. This undergoes cleavage with a nuclease and some base modification:
- CCA is added to the 3' end of each tRNA.
- Bases in rRNA may be methylated.
- Bases in tRNA may be modified to produce inosine, pseudouridine, and dihydrouridine.

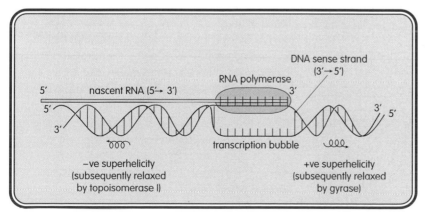

Fig. 5.26 RNA chain elongation. The RNA molecule develops in a straight line while DNA rotates. (Adapted with permission from *Biochemistry* by Dr D.Voet and Dr J.C. Voet, John Wiley & Sons, 1990.)

Transcription of eukaryotic RNA				
Name	**Site of synthesis**	**Polymerase responsible**	**Features of promoter sequence**	**Features of RNA molecules**
hnRNA	nucleoplasm	Pol II	long and diverse; housekeeping genes contain a GC box; structural genes contain a TATA box	precursors of mRNA: mature mRNA produced by splicing
tRNA	nucleoplasm	Pol III	within transcribed region of gene	clover-leaf structure produced by secondary structure
rRNA	nucleolus (except 5 S—synthesized in the nucleoplasm	Pol I for 5.8, 18, 28 S; Pol III for 5 S	Pol I promoter extends from −142 to +6 of RNA; genes −7 to +6 guide Pol I to the initiation site	complex with proteins to form ribosomes
snRNA	nucleoplasm			forms complexes called snRNPs (or snurps; see p. 90) associated with the formation of spliceosomes for post-transcriptional modification of hnRNA
mt-mRNA	mitochondrion	mitochondrion-specific polymerase		associated with protein synthesis in the mitochondria
mt-tRNA	mitochondrion	mitochondrion-specific polymerase		associated with protein synthesis in the mitochondria

Fig. 5.27 Transcription of eukaryotic RNA. (A, adenine; C, cytosine; G, guanine; sn, small nuclear; hn, heterogeneous nuclear; mt, mitochondrial; sn, T, thymine; snRNP, small nuclear ribonucleoproteins.)

DNA replication versus RNA transcription:
- **Both are semi-conservative.**
- **Primer is required to initiate DNA replication and the initiation complex initiates transcription.**
- **Template is conserved in transcription, but not in DNA replication.**

Eukaryotic transcription

The different classes of RNA involved in eukaryotic RNA transcription are listed in Fig. 5.27.

Sequence of events
Initiation
The process of initiation is illustrated in Fig. 5.28.

Elongation
The overall equation is the same as for prokaryotic elongation. α-amanitin is a potent inhibitor of RNA Pol II and a weak inhibitor of Pol III. It comes from the poisonous death cap mushroom *Amanita phalloides*. It specifically blocks the elongation step of Pol II and Pol III, so has been a useful tool in mechanistic studies. In humans, 5–6 mg of α-amanitin can be fatal. Death is usually from liver failure several days after ingestion of the poison.

Termination
This is a far less precise process in eukaryotes than in prokaryotes because the 3′ end of the molecule undergoes post-transcriptional modification where the transcript is cleaved at a highly conserved AAUAAA sequence. Transcription can sometimes carry on for hundreds of bases past this site. The precise signal for termination of transcription has not yet been found.

Eukaryotic post-transcriptional modification
Addition of a 5′ cap
This is a very early modification that occurs soon after

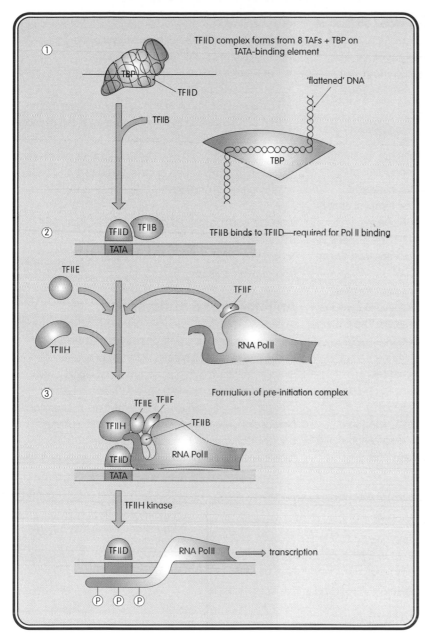

① TFIID complex forms from 8 TAFs + TBP on TATA-binding element

TBP

TFIID

TFIIB

'flattened' DNA

TBP

② TFIID TFIIB

TATA

TFIIB binds to TFIID—required for Pol II binding

TFIIE

TFIIF

TFIIH

RNA PolII

③ Formation of pre-initiation complex

TFIIE TFIIF

TFIIH

TFIIB

TFIID

RNA PolII

TATA

TFIIH kinase

TFIID

RNA PolII → transcription

P P P

Fig. 5.28 Initiation of transcription with eukaryotic RNA polymerase II. In the final stage, TFIIH phosphorylates amino acids in the tail of RNA Pol II, which reduces its affinity for TAFs and releases RNA Pol II for transcription. (A, adenine; T, thymine; TAF, TATA-associated factor; TBP, TATA -binding protein—a saddle-shaped protein that unwinds the DNA helix; TF, transcription factor). (Adapted with permission from *The Journal of Molecular Biology* **150**: 92–120., by J. Engel, E. Odermatt, A. Engel, J.A. Madr and H. Furthmayr *et al.* 1981.)(Courtesy of H. Furthymayr.)

transcription initiation. A cap structure containing 7-methylguanosine is enzymatically added to the 5′ end of the growing transcript. It is thought to have three functions :

• It protects the mRNA from enzymatic attack.
• It aids in splicing.
• It enhances translation of the mRNA.

The eukaryotic genome is larger than the prokaryotic genome, so it needs more RNA polymerases to read a greater variety of genes.

89

3′ cleavage at the AAUAAA sequence and addition of a poly(A) tail

The cleavage gives the 3′ end of the transcript a well-defined end. The poly(A) tail is generated from adenosine triphosphate (ATP) by the enzyme poly(A) polymerase.

Splicing

Heterogeneous nuclear RNAs (hnRNAs) are the primary transcripts from genomic DNA. The production of mature eukaryotic mRNAs from hnRNA involves a process called gene splicing. This is the removal of non-coding introns and the joining together of the intervening exons. This process occurs in the nucleus in an RNA–protein complex called the spliceosome. Each spliceosome consists of:

- A core structure made up of three subunits called snRNPs (pronounced 'snurps'). Each snRNP contains at least one snRNA and several proteins. The protein subunits are named after the associated snRNAs, U1, U2, and [U4/U6, U5].
- Non-snurp splicing factors and an hnRNA.

The splicing process relies on the existence of consensus sequences within the hnRNA, which are recognized by the spliceosome. Each intron begins with a 5′-GU and ends with AG-3′, and these sites are recognized by the snRNAs; for example U1 binds to the 5′ splice site and U2 binds to the branch site. The process consists of the following stages :

- Cut 5′ splice site.
- Cut 3′ splice site.
- Release of the intron by formation of a lariat loop (Fig. 5.29) between the 5′ splice site and the 'branch site' in the centre of the intron.
- Joining together of exons by transesterification—the free -OH group of one exon is linked to the free 5′ phosphate of another.

Comparison of prokaryotic and eukaryotic transcription

A comparison of prokaryotic and eukaryotic transcription is shown in Fig. 5.30.

Antibiotics and transcription

Actinomycin inhibits both RNA and DNA polymerases by intercalating between G–C pairs in duplex DNA to inhibit nucleic acid synthesis. Rifampicin specifically inhibits prokaryotic RNA polymerases. It blocks chain elongation by remaining bound to the promoter to prevent new initiation complexes forming. It does not block eukaryotic RNA polymerases so it is a useful bactericidal agent against Gram-positive bacteria and tuberculosis.

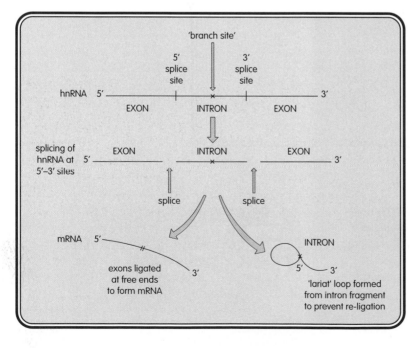

Fig. 5.29 Processes of intron excision from hnRNA to produce the mRNA strand which may be used for translation

Comparison of prokaryotic and eukaryotic transcription		
	Prokaryotic	**Eukaryotic**

site of transcription	cytoplasm	nucleus:
		5.8 S/18 S/28 S rRNA
		  in nucleolus
		5 S rRNA, tRNA, mRNA
		  in nucleoplasm

RNA polymerase	single species: RNAP (*E. coli*); large holoenzyme; core enzyme consists of four subunits: $\alpha_2\beta\beta'$	three RNA polymerases in nucleus: Pol I transcribes rRNA; Pol II, mRNA; Pol III, rRNA and tRNA; consist of two large subunits with homology to the prokaryotic β subunits and a complex array of approximately 12 small subunits (e.g. Pol II assembly initiated by TFIID binding to promoter)
initiation	S subunit associates with the core enzyme and facilitates binding to the promoter	complex assembly of proteins
termination	RNA forms stable hairpin loop between A–T-rich and G–C-rich region, then weak base pairing between poly(U) RNA and DNA encourages dissociation; the ρ factor is an enzyme that facilitates transcription termination with or without the hairpin loop	termination is imprecise and signal is unknown
post-transcriptional modification	mRNA requires little or no modification	hnRNA = mRNA precursor: 5′ methyl cap added during transcription; 3′ end cleaved at AAUAAA site and poly(A) tail added; introns removed by splicing
mRNA	polycistronic: each transcript can code for more than one polypeptide	monocistronic: can code for only one polypeptide

- ⊚ **Define transcription and translation.**
- ⊚ **Explain the initiation, elongation, and termination of prokaryotic transcription (include its modification) and eukaryotic transcription (include splicing).**
- ⊚ **Describe how α-amantin, actinomycin, and rifampicin exert their antibiotic effects.**
- ⊚ **Compare prokaryotic and eukaryotic processes of transcription.**

GENETIC CODE

Coding properties of nucleic acids

In the translation process from DNA to protein, amino acids are coded for by groups of three bases called codons. Since nucleic acids contain four bases, codons could specify 4^3 (64) amino acids.

Properties of the genetic code

The properties of the genetic code are as follows:

- Redundancy. Since there are 64 codons and only 20 amino acids commonly used in polypeptide synthesis, a large proportion of the codons can be considered redundant.
- Degeneracy. The genetic code is degenerate, which means that more than one codon codes for each amino acid. This reduces the amount of redundancy.
- Code degeneracy invokes the wobble hypothesis. Non-Watson–Crick base pairing sometimes occurs between the codon and the third base on the tRNA anti-codon (Fig. 5.31). This occurs more frequently when the third base is modified by altering base–base interactions.
- The code is non-overlapping and comma free.
- Universality. The same genetic code is seen in almost all living organisms.
- Stop codons or 'nonsense triplets' mark the end of a polypeptide. They signal to the ribosome to stop protein synthesis.

The standard genetic code is shown in Fig. 5.32.

Structure of genes

A gene is a nucleotide coding sequence that results in the production of a functional mRNA and polypeptide. The 'one gene, one polypeptide' hypothesis states that the base sequence of DNA determines the amino acid sequence in the corresponding polypeptide.

Exons are expressed sequences (i.e. ones that code for amino acids) and introns are the non-coding intervening sequences. Introns are:

- Rare in prokaryotic genes.
- Uncommon in lower eukaryotes such as yeast.
- Abundant in higher eukaryotes (vertebrate structural genes rarely lack introns).

The promoter region lies in the DNA immediately preceding a gene. Sequence analysis studies have revealed 'consensus' sequences in prokaryotes and eukaryotes, which are vital for promoter function. The most conserved sequence in the *E.coli* promoter is the TATAAT box, which forms the initial binding site for the

Allowed wobble pairings in the third codon–anticodon position	
5'-anticodon base	3'-codon base
C	G
A	U
U	A or G
G	U or C
I	U, C or A

Fig. 5.31 Wobble hypothesis. (A, adenine; C, cytosine; G, guanine; I, inosine; T, thymine; U, uracil.)

Standard genetic code				
first position (5' end)	second	position		third position (3' end)
	U	C	A	G	
U	Phe	Ser	Tyr	Cys	U
U	Phe	Ser	Tyr	Cys	C
U	Leu	Ser	Stop	Stop	A
U	Leu	Ser	Stop	Trp	G
C	Leu	Pro	His	Arg	U
C	Leu	Pro	His	Arg	C
C	Leu	Pro	Gln	Arg	A
C	Leu	Pro	Gln	Arg	G
A	Ile	Thr	Asn	Ser	U
A	Ile	Thr	Asn	Ser	C
A	Ile	Thr	Lys	Arg	A
A	Met	Thr	Lys	Arg	G
G	Val	Ala	Asp	Gly	U
G	Val	Ala	Asp	Gly	C
G	Val	Ala	Glu	Gly	A
G	Val	Ala	Glu	Gly	G

the standard genetic code. (A, adenine; C, cytosine; G, guanine; T, thymine; U, uracil)

Fig. 5.32 Standard genetic code. (A, adenine; C, cytosine; G, guanine; T, thymine; U, uracil.) To find out which amino acid a particular codon codes for, first select the 5' end base. Then read across to select the column corresponding to the second position base. Read down to find the 3' end base and locate the row on which the corresponding amino acid lies.

transcription enzyme RNAP. The situation is more complex in eukaryotes. More consensus sequences have been detected and include the GC box (GGGCGG), the TATA box, and the CAAT box. Each region has been shown to bind specific transcription factors—proteins involved in the regulation of gene expression (see Fig. 5.28). The promoter region is 'polar' as it acts in one direction only to control the gene it precedes. It determines the start site for gene expression.

Eukaryotic cells also have enhancer regions, which can occur anywhere before, after, or within a gene. They are thought to affect the activity of their cognate promoter. Interaction between enhancer and promoter elements exerts a hierarchical control over gene expression that is precise and specific (Fig. 5.33).

Clusters of related genes can occur in the human genome. They arise from the duplication of a primitive precursor and share similar intron–exon patterns. The HLA (human leucocyte antigen) complex on the short arm of chromosome 6 is an example of a gene cluster. The term haplotype describes a cluster of alleles (alleles are alternative versions of a gene) that occur together on a DNA segment and are inherited together. The HLA haplotype genes:

- Are mostly members of the immunoglobulin superfamily—a family of hundreds of genes, which occur throughout the human genome and are involved in cell surface recognition.
- Share sets of related exons, which indicates that they have evolved from an ancestral gene by duplication.
- Are characterized by the presence of immunoglobulin 'domains' (or folds) consisting of 110 amino acid residues stabilized by a disulphide bridge.

There are three classes of HLA genes. Classes I and II are also known as the histocompatibility or transplant rejection genes as they are responsible for organ transplant rejection (Fig. 5.34).

Mitochondrial DNA

Mitochondria contain their own DNA, which differs from that in the rest of the cell. Human mitochondrial DNA consists of 16 569 base pairs of circular dsDNA. It codes for:

- 22 mitochondrial (mt) tRNAs
- Two mt rRNAs.
- 13 proteins synthesized by the mitochondrion's own protein-synthesizing machinery. All are subunits of the oxidative phosphorylation pathway.

The differences between mitochondrial DNA code and nuclear DNA code are shown in Fig. 5.35. Mitochondrial DNA code is simpler and more degenerate, probably because it can afford to be more tolerant of changes than nuclear DNA because of its smaller size. Codon/anticodon pairings show more 'wobble' pairings than in the process originating in the nucleus. This is made possible by unusual mt tRNA sequences such as mt tRNA^{ser}, which lacks a D arm.

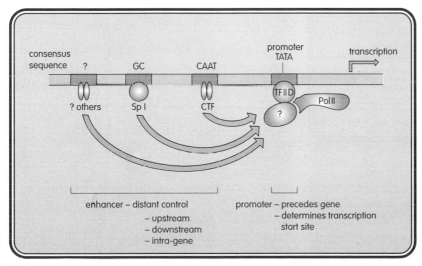

Fig. 5.33 Hierarchical control over gene expression in eukaryotes. There is sequence homology between TATAAT and eukaryotic TATA. Both form the site of the transcription initiation complex. (A, adenine; T, thymine; C, cytosine; G, guanine.)

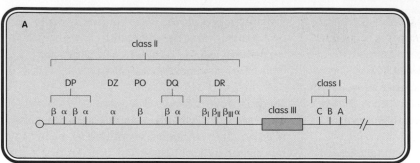

Fig. 5.34 (A) Diagram to illustrate the classification of human leucocyte antigen (HLA) haplotype genes. (B) Features of different classes of HLA genes. **<60>**

Classification of the HLA haplotype genes			
	Class I	**Class II**	**Class III**
main products	A, B, C code for α_1, α_2, α_3 proteins, which complex with β_2 microglobulin coded for on chromosome 15	DR, DP, DQ	complement components C4a, C4b, TNF, etc
expressed	on surface of all cells except erythrocytes	by antigen-presenting cells (e.g. macrophages and B lymphocytes)	
structure		each has an α and a β domain	sequence homologies with class I and class II

Fig. 5.35 Summary of variations between mitochondrial and standard genetic code. (N, one of four nucleotides.)

Variations between mitochondrial and standard genetic code		
	Standard	**Mammalian mitochondrion**
UGA	Stop	Trp
AUA	Ile	Met (initiation signal)
CUN	Leu	–
AGA/AGG	Arg	Stop
CGG	Arg	–

- Explain what is meant by a codon.
- Explain 'code degeneracy' and the 'wobble hypothesis'.
- Draw a diagrammatic representation of a eukaryotic gene.
- Describe what are mitochondrial DNA codes and how they differ from nuclear DNA.

TRANSLATION AND PROTEIN SYNTHESIS

Protein synthesis in prokaryotes

The components needed for translation are mRNA, tRNA, ribosome, GTP, initiation factors, elongation factors.

Aminoacyl transferase

Amino acid + tRNA $\quad \rightarrow \quad$ Aminoacyl-tRNA

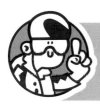

Learn this equation, it often comes up in examinations.

   Amino acids combine with their corresponding tRNA in a reaction catalysed by a specific aminoacyl transferase. This incorporates a high-energy ester bond between the aminoacyl group and the 3' CCA group of the tRNA. The energy released when this bond is broken drives the peptide bond formation step of chain elongation. Translation consists of three stages initiation, elongation, and termination (see transcription, p. 86).

Initiation

The initiation complex is composed of a ribosome, mRNA, and initiator tRNA. The process of initiation requires:

- Three initiation factors, IF-1, IF-2, and IF-3.
- A molecule of GTP.

Initiator tRNA is f-Met–tRNA. It carries a formylated methionine residue and recognizes an AUG codon on the mRNA. Each mRNA contains many AUG codons in its various reading frames. The one corresponding to the start of translation is preceded by a purine-rich tract of nucleotides called the Shine–Dalgarno sequence. This binds to a corresponding pyrimidine-rich sequence in the rIbosomal S unit (Fig. 5.36).

Note that IF stands for 'initiation factor', EF stands for 'elongation factor', and RF stands for 'release factor.'

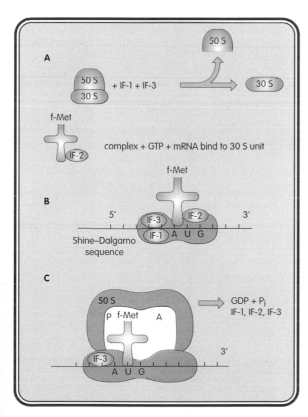

Fig. 5.36 Initiation factors of prokaryotic translation. (A) IF-1 and IF-3 bind to 30 S subunit of ribosome to promote dissociation of 50 S subunit. (B) f-Met-IF-2 complex and GTP and mRNA bind to 30 S unit. IF-2 is required for f-Met-tRNA binding to mRNA. f-Met-tRNA–mRNA binding is not therefore dependent upon codon–anti-codon association. IF-3 assists ribosomal binding to the Shine–Dalgarno sequence on mRNA. (C) IF-3 is released and GTP hydrolysed. The 50 S subunit associates and IF-1 and IF-2 are released. f-Met-tRNA lies in the P site so the A site is ready to accept incoming tRNA. (Note that f-Met-tRNA is the only tRNA that does not enter the ribosome via the A site.)

The Molecular Basis of Genetics

Elongation

Chain elongation involves the addition of aminoacyl residues to the growing polypeptide. It is a three-stage process.

Step one

Aminoacyl-tRNA binds to the ribosomal A site (Fig. 5.37) as follows:

- Complex of aminoacyl-tRNA, GTP, and EF-Tu is formed.
- Codon–anticodon binding with concomitant hydrolysis of GTP.
- Release of GDP and inorganic phosphate (P_i) and EF-Tu.

Step two

Peptide bond formation is catalysed by a peptidyl transferase in the 50 S subunit. Peptidyl group in the P site is added onto the aminoacyl group in the A site. The reaction is driven by a high-energy ester bond between the aminoacyl group and tRNA (see p. 95.)

Step three

The translocation (Fig. 5.38) process occurs as follows:

- Uncharged tRNA is expelled.
- Peptidyl-tRNA is transferred from the A site to the P site. This requires EF-G and GTP.
- The tRNA is still bound to the mRNA codon, so, as the peptidyl-tRNA moves across from the A site to the P site, the mRNA moves with it. A new codon now lies in the A site. This mechanism allows the reading frame to be maintained.

In an *E. coli* cell almost all tRNAs are sequestered by EF-Tu—this is vital for translation to occur because EF-Tu-tRNA association is the rate-limiting step of the translation process.

Termination

The termination codons, UAA, UAG, and UGA are recognized by release factors rather than tRNAs:

- RF-1 recognizes UAA and UAG.
- RF-2 recognizes UAA and UGA.
- RF-3, which binds GTP, stimulates ribosomal binding of RF-1 and RF-2.

The binding of an RF causes the peptidyl transferase to transfer the peptidyl group to water rather than to an aminoacyl group. This results in the release of a free polypeptide. The uncharged tRNA is released from the ribosome and the RFs are expelled.

Protein synthesis in eukaryotes

Protein synthesis is very similar in eukaryotes, but more associated factors are involved. Fig. 5.39 compares prokaryotic and eukaryotic translation.

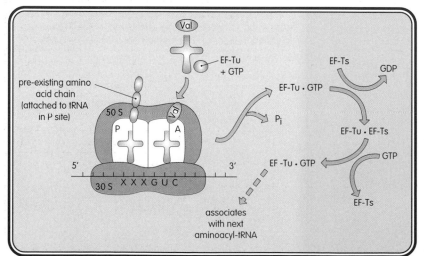

Fig. 5.37 Step one of chain elongation: aminoacyl-tRNA binding to ribosomal A site. Elongation factors EF-Tu + EF-Ts interact to liberate EF-Tu which can then associate with another free aminoacyl-tRNA. GTP is hydrolyzed to GDP + P_i during this recycling process

Endoplasmic reticulum

Endoplasmic reticulum (ER) is a diffuse system of membrane-bound cisternae in the cytoplasm of eukaryotic cells (see Chapter 1). There are two types—rough endoplasmic reticulum (RER) and smooth endoplasmic reticulum (SER). The membranes of RER have ribosomes attached to them and are specialized for the synthesis and secretion of proteins. The SER is devoid of ribosomes. It is responsible for the synthesis of cholesterol and phospholipids and is prominent in cells that are active in lipid biosynthesis such as liver cells.

Proteins bound for organelles, plasma membrane, or export enter the ER lumen as they are translated following interactions between specific proteins on the ribosome, ER membrane, and in the cytoplasm (see pp.100–101).

Control of protein synthesis
Sites of regulation of protein synthesis

Control of protein synthesis is synonymous with control of gene expression. In the prokaryote, control can be at the level of transcription or translation. The situation is

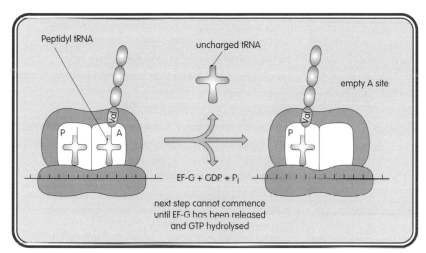

Fig. 5.38 Step three of chain elongation: translocation. Unchanged tRNA is expelled from the A site and the peptidyl-tRNA is transferred from the A site to the P site.

	Comparison between prokaryotic and eukaryotic translation	
	Prokaryotes	**Eukaryotes**
ribosome	large subunit 50 S, small subunit 30 S, whole ribosome 70 S	large subunit 60 S, small subunit 40 S, whole ribosome 80 S
initiation	three initiation factors called IF-1, 2, 3; initiator tRNA carries f-Met (formylated methionine); start codon AUG; Shine–Dalgarno sequence precedes the start site on the mRNA; binds to a complementary sequence on the ribosome's S subunit	over 10 initiation factors with multiple subunits called eIFs ('e' for eukaryote); initiator tRNA carries Met (not N-formylated); start codon AUG; no Shine–Dalgarno sequence; mRNA 5'-methylated cap may have a binding site on ribosome S subunit to guide translation complex to start site
type of mRNA code	polycistronic (mRNA often codes for more than one protein)	monocistronic (mRNA always codes for a single protein)
elongation	elongation factors called EF-Tu, EF-Ts and EF-G	EF-Tu and EF-Ts are replaced by a single factor, eEF-1; EF-G replaced by eEF-2
termination	three release factors, RF-1, 2, 3: RF-3 is bound to GTP and the RF-3–GTP complex stimulates ribosomal binding of RF-1 and 2; GTP hydrolysis triggers complex to disassemble	single release factor, eRF, which binds to the ribosome with GTP; GTP hydrolysis triggers eRF release from ribosome

Fig. 5.39 Comparison between prokaryotic and eukaryotic translation.

more complex in eukaryotes and a total of six control points have been identified (Fig. 5.40).

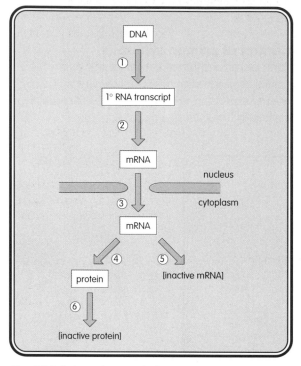

Fig. 5.40 Eukaryotic control of gene expression. (1) Transcription control. (2) Processing of transcript. (3) Transport control. (4) Translational control by selection of ribosomes by mRNA. (5) mRNA degradation control. (6) Protein activity control and post-translational modification.

Elongation factors and bacterial toxins

EFs are vital to the process of translation. For example the *E. coli* factor EF-Tu controls the rate-limiting step of translation. In the cytoplasm of normal *E. coli* cells every aminoacyl-tRNA is sequestered by an EF-Tu protein. In the absence of this factor the rate of protein synthesis is too slow to support cell growth.

Translation can be blocked by bacterial toxins. The toxin produced by *Corynebacterium diphtheriae* (the organism causing diphtheria), for example, inhibits translation by inactivating EF-2.

Antibiotics and protein synthesis

Many antibiotics block protein synthesis, either by blocking translation or by other means. Some are particularly useful therapeutically because they specifically target prokaryote translation (see Fig. 5.41).

Antibiotics and mitochondria

The translation process in eukaryotic mitochondria is very similar to that in prokaryotes. Antibiotics that inhibit prokaryotic protein synthesis can also affect mitochondrial protein synthesis. Antibiotics, however, do not harm their mammalian host because:

- Some antibiotics are unable to cross the inner mitochondrial membrane.
- Mitochondria are replaced at cell division. This occurs relatively slowly in most cells so mitochondria are depleted only with long-term antibiotic use.
- In rapidly dividing cells the local environment can

Fig. 5.41 Antibiotics that inhibit translation.

Antibiotics that inhibit translation		
Antibiotic	**Site of action**	**Process inhibited**
streptomycin	prokaryote ribosomal 30 S subunit	initiation/elongation (causes mRNA misreading)
erythromycin	prokaryote 50 S subunit	translocation
chloramphenicol	prokaryote 50 S subunit	peptidyl transferase
cycloheximide	eukaryote 60 S subunit	peptidyl transferase
tetracycline	prokaryote 30 S subunit	aminoacyl tRNA binding to ribosome A site
puromycin	ribosome	peptide transfer causes premature termination as it mimics an aminoacyl tRNA

sometimes prevent uptake of antibiotic (e.g. in bone, high calcium levels cause the formation of calcium–tetracycline so the drug cannot be taken up by cells in the bone marrow).

Constitutive, inducible, and repressible enzymes

Constitutive enzymes are present at fixed concentrations in the cell, irrespective of changes in the cell environment. They are examples of products of housekeeping genes.

The level of expression of inducible/repressible enzymes is altered by the cellular environment. A certain chemical may induce the expression of a gene, while another chemical may repress its expression. Enzyme induction can be a side effect of drug treatments that cause important drug

interactions, for example, treatment with phenytoin and warfarin. Phenytoin is a liver enzyme inducer and causes increased levels of the enzyme system that metabolizes warfarin, so if the drugs are taken together the warfarin is rapidly metabolized and high doses are required to keep it in the therapeutic range. Subsequent withdrawal of the phenytoin will cause the enzyme induction to cease and can cause a rebound haemorrhage due to the massively increased systemic levels of warfarin.

Operons and enzyme induction/repression

An operon is a cluster of genes in bacterial DNA that is transcribed from one promoter to give a polycistronic mRNA. The 'lac operon' in E. coli has been particularly well studied and codes for three genes involved in the metabolism of lactose (Fig. 5.42).

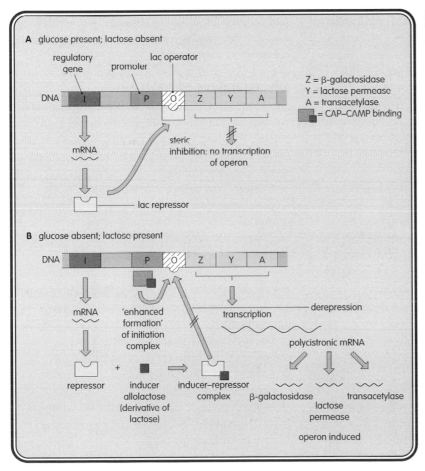

Fig. 5.42 The *lac* operon. (A) The '*lac* repressor' binds to the '*lac* operator' with great affinity. The *lac* operator is formed by a stretch of DNA that overlaps with the operon's initiation site. *Lac* repressor binding prevents the formation of a transcription initiation complex so transcription cannot occur. (B) Lactose binds to the *lac* repressor and changes its shape so it has a much lower affinity for the *lac* operator, and derepression occurs. An initiation complex forms and transcription begins. At the same time, low levels of glucose cause an increase in intracellular cAMP, which binds to catabolite activator protein (CAP). The CAP–cAMP complex binds to the *lac* operon promoter region and encourages the formation of an RNA initiation complex. (A, Y, Z, are genes for transacetylase, lactose permease, β-galactosidase, respectively).

POST-TRANSLATIONAL MODIFICATION OF PROTEINS

Concepts

Post-translational modification is the alteration of proteins after translation. These alterations include:

- Peptide cleavage.
- Covalent modifications such as glycosylation, phosphorylation, carboxylation, and hydroxylation of specific residues.

The modifications give proteins functional activity.

A newly synthesized protein can be destined for secretion, the cytoplasm, extracellular, membrane, lysosome, or another organelle. Various signals within the protein (the signal peptide) or non-protein subunits (added by post-translational modification) help the protein to reach its destination.

Signal peptide

This is not strictly related to post-translational modification, but it is involved in a process vital to it. The signal peptide has already been mentioned above. It is responsible for translocating developing polypeptides destined for extracellular secretion, membrane, lysosomes, and other organelles, into the ER lumen as

All proteins are translocated into the ER lumen except those destined for the cytoplasm.

they are translated (Fig. 5.43). The signal peptide is near the amino terminus of the polypeptide and contains hydrophobic residues such as phenylalanine.

Inside the ER lumen the polypeptide can undergo post-translational modifications specific to each protein. Proteins destined for extracellular secretion are transported to the Golgi apparatus in vesicles, which bud off the ER. Further modification may take place here and the secretory protein is packaged into vesicles that fuse with the cell plasma membrane, releasing their contents to the exterior.

Glycosylation of proteins

This occurs in the ER lumen or the Golgi apparatus and involves the addition of an oligosaccharide to a specific residue. There are two types of glycosylation, designated *N*-linked and *O*-linked, and the saccharide is added by a specific glycosyltransferase:

- *N*-linked—the oligosaccharide is added to the polypeptide by a β-*N*-glycosidic bond to an Asp residue.
- *O*-linked—the oligosaccharide is an α-*O*-glycosidic bond to a Ser or Thr residue.

The oligosaccharide is carried on a lipid-soluble carrier. It is then transferred to a specific residue on the targeted protein.

Glycosylation is important for correct compartmentalization of proteins within the cell:

- *O*-linked glycosylation is involved in the production of blood group antigens.
- *N*-linked glycosylation is involved in the transfer of acid hydrolase to lysosomes and the production of mature antibodies.

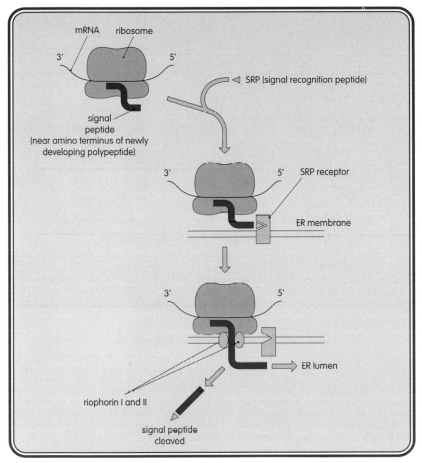

Fig. 5.43 Role of the signal peptide in translocation into the ER lumen. The signal peptide. is near the amino terminus of the newly developing polypeptide. It associates with a cytoplasmic signal recognition peptide (SRP) and then with an SRP receptor ('docking protein') on the ER membrane. The ribosome then interlocks between two membrane-associated proteins, riophorin I and II, which drive the developing polypeptide into the ER lumen.

Other modification of proteins

Proteins may be modified by:

- Phosphorylation, which targets Ser or Tyr residues and tends to regulate enzyme activity (Ser) or protein activity (Tyr). Kinases transfer phosphate groups from ATP onto the target residue.
- Sulphation, which targets Tyr. It is important in compartmentalization (e.g. marking proteins for export) and biological activity.
- Hydroxylation, which targets Lys and Pro residues. It is very important in the production of collagen (and extracellular matrix protein). The hydroxylation of Lys and Pro residues occurs during translation and is essential for the formation of the collagen triple helix.
- Lipidation of Cys and Gly residues, which is necessary for anchoring proteins such as antibody receptors into the membrane.

- Acetylation of Lys, which can change the charge of the residue. In histone H4, this alters its binding properties to DNA.
- Cleavage, which activates some enzymes and hormones.

Fig. 5.44 summarizes post-translational modifications.

Disorders of post-translational modification

I-cell disease is a storage disease characterized by psychomotor retardation, skeletal deformation, and early death. It results from a deficiency of mannose-6-phosphate glycosyltransferase, which is responsible for glycosylation of enzymes destined for lysosomes. The enzymes lack their recognition markers so are secreted into the extracellular matrix rather than being taken up by lysosomes.

Summary of some post-translational modifications				
Destination	Protein function	Modification	Residue	Example
secreted	structural	hydroxylation	Lys/Pro	collagen
	enzyme	hydrolytic cleavage	(peptide bond)	pepsinogen → pepsin
	hormone	hydrolytic cleavage	(peptide bond)	proinsulin → insulin
	clotting factor	carboxylation	Glu	prothrombin → thrombin
	antibody	glycosylation (N-linked)	Asp	IgG
membrane	receptor	lipidation	Gly/Cys	antibody receptors
	cell recognition	glycosylation (O-linked)	Ser	blood group antigens
	receptor activation	phosphorylation	Tyr	growth factor receptor activation
cytoplasm	enzyme	phosphorylation	Tyr	activation
lysosome	hydrolytic enzymes	glycosylation (N-linked)	Asp	acid hydrolases

Fig. 5.44 Summary of some post-translational modifications.

- Explain what is meant by post-translational modification.
- Explain the role of the signal peptide.
- Describe modification by glycosylation, with examples.
- Describe other methods of modification, with examples.
- Give an example of a disorder of post-translational modification.

GENETICS OF BACTERIA AND VIRUSES

Bacterial genetics.

There are fundamental differences between bacterial and mammalian cells and, as a result, some chemicals that are toxic to bacteria can be tolerated by mammals. Antimicrobial agents can be taken by humans in appropriate amounts to treat bacterial infections without harming the host. (NB An antibiotic is an antimicrobial agent manufactured by living organisms rather than by chemical synthesis). A summary of the differences between bacterial and human cells is given in Fig. 5.45.

Antimicrobial agents
Inhibitors of nucleic acid synthesis
These agents:

- Target the folic acid synthesis pathway. (This pathway produces tetrahydrofolate, which is essential for base synthesis.)
- Do not affect mammalian cells because mammals obtain folic acid from their diet.
- Are bacteriostatic— they halt bacterial growth but do not kill them.

Sulphonamides (e.g. sulphadiazine) are analogues of γ-aminobenzoic acid. Trimethoprim inhibits dihydrofolate reductase. It is used in the treatment of urinary tract infections.

Inhibitors of DNA gyrase
Quinolones (e.g. ciprofloxacin) inhibit DNA gyrase, the enzyme which causes DNA unwinding. They are bactericidal—they kill bacteria.

Differences between bacterial and human cells		
	Bacterial	**Human**
form of genetic material	prokaryotic, no nucleus or nucleolus, single DNA thread tightly coiled by topoisomerases, extra-chromosomal elements called plasmids, double stranded	eukaryotic, linear DNA, associated with proteins to form chromosomes, double stranded
cell size	average diameter 0.5–5 μm	up to 40 μm
protein synthesis	ribosomal subunits 50 S and 30 S	subunits 60 S and 40 S
nucleic acid synthesis	folate must be synthesized *de novo* for base synthesis	folate can be obtained from the diet
organelles	few, associated with respiration and photosynthesis	many and diverse

Fig. 5.45 Summary of the differences between bacterial and human cells.

Inhibitors of cell wall synthesis

The bacterial cell wall is rigid and contains linear peptidoglycans, which are crosslinked by peptides. An important group of antimicrobials disrupt cell wall synthesis by inhibiting formation of crosslinks. They all contain a β-lactam ring that gives them their antimicrobial activity. They are bactericidal and are not effective against Gram-negative bacteria because they cannot penetrate the phospholipid-rich outer membrane.

Penicillins were the first group of antibiotics to be discovered and are still important clinically. Benzylpenicillin:

- Is used in the treatment of pneumococcal, streptococcal, and meningococcal infections.
- Is not effective orally so is given by injection.

Cephalosporins have a similar spectrum to penicillin, although individual agents are active against certain bacteria. Cefuroxime is used prophylactically in surgery. It is active against *Staphylococcus aureus* (Gram positive) and is resistant to bacterial β-lactamase. Ceftazidime is active against *Pseudomonas aeruginosa*, which can cause infections in immunosuppressed patients.

Inhibitors of protein synthesis

These have already been mentioned on p.98. They target prokaryotic ribosomes (50 S L subunit and 30 S S subunit) and do not affect mammalian ribosomes (60 S L subunit and 40 S S subunit).

Transfer of genetic material

The bacterial genome is haploid: there is only one complete set of genetic material. Genetic material can be transferred between bacteria to produce partial zygotes and the three mechanisms of genetic transfer between bacteria are:

- Transformation—certain bacteria release DNA into the environment that can be taken up by other bacteria by a receptor uptake mechanism. If the DNA is compatible, it is incorporated into the bacterial genome; otherwise, it is degraded by exonucleases.
- Transduction—a fragment of bacterial DNA is incorporated into a bacteriophage during assembly. (Bacteriophages are viruses that infect bacteria). One in 10^6 bacteriophages contains bacterial DNA and when it infects the next bacterium, the viral genome and the bacterial DNA are introduced into the new host cell. Again, if the bacterial DNA is compatible it can be integrated into the host's genome.
- Conjugation—the bacterial form of sexual reproduction. Two strains of bacteria exist; F positive (F^+) and F negative (F^-). F positive cells possess a plasmid (extra-chromosomal piece of genetic material) called the F factor. F^+ cells possess a pilus (a cytoplasmic projection) which gives them the ability to attach to other bacterial cells via cytoplasmic bridges through which genetic material can be transferred. This process is called conjugation (Fig. 5.46)

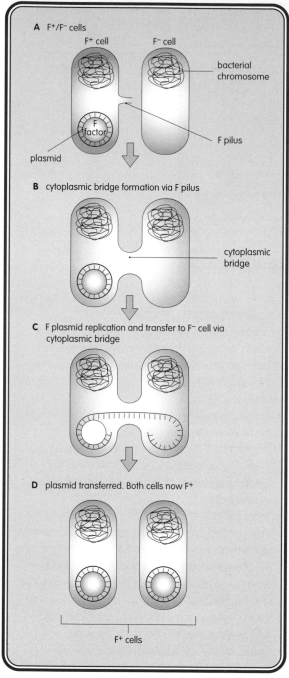

Fig. 5.46 Bacterial conjugation. (A) The ability to conjugate is conferred by a plasmid called the F factor. Bacteria with the plasmid are F+. (B) F+ cells contain thread-like projections called F pili and can attach to F− cells to form a cytoplasmic bridge. (C) F plasmid is replicated and a single stranded replica is transferred along the bridge. (D) Within the recipient, the transferred material is replicated to form a new plasmid.

Sometimes the F factor becomes incorporated into the bacterial genome to create high frequency of recombinations (Hfr) cells. During conjugation all of the bacterial DNA is replicated (the F factor creates the starting point for replication). The replicated DNA is passed along the cytoplasmic bridge into the recipient cell. Variable amounts of DNA are transferred because the bridge invariably breaks down before the process has been completed. Parts of the newly introduced DNA are then incorporated into the recipient genome.

The conjugation process is another way for prokaryotes to 'mix up' their gene pool and adapt to their environment; for example, it can produce antibiotic-resistant strains of bacteria such as the multiply resistant strain of enterococci that has evolved as a result of using antibiotics in cattle feed. Methicillin-resistant *S. aureus* (MRSA) is a threat in hospital wards as it can spread very rapidly among ill patients and is very hard to eradicate.

Viral genetics

Viruses are infectious particles consisting of a nucleic acid enclosed in a protein coat called the capsid, which may or may not be surrounded by a phospholipid envelope. They adsorb onto the surface of susceptible cells and inject their nucleic acid. They are ultimate parasites as they have no metabolism of their own and rely entirely on their host for replication and production of new virus particles. They contain either DNA or RNA, never both. The life cycle of a virus has ten stages (Fig. 5.47).

DNA viruses

The viral DNA is transcribed into mRNA using host RNA polymerase (in the nucleus). The mRNA diffuses into the cytoplasm, associates with ribosomes, and is translated into viral proteins. These are either:

- Structural and are used to assemble new virions (individual virus particles).
- Non-structural, mainly enzymes involved in replication of the viral genome.

Details of some important DNA viruses are given in Fig. 5.48.

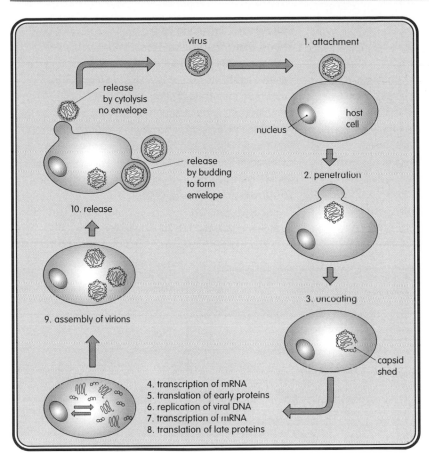

Fig. 5.47 Life cycle of a virus, showing ten different stages.

Fig. 5.48 Some important DNA viruses.

Class	Family	Species	Disease
double stranded DNA	Papovaviridae	papillomavirus	human warts
	Adenoviridae	adenovirus	pharyngitis, acute respiratory disease, acute gastroenteritis
	Herpesviridae	herpes simplex (HSV)	cold sores (type I), genital herpes (type II)
		varicella zoster virus (VZV)	chickenpox (varicella), shingles (zoster)
		Epstein–Barr (EBV)	glandular fever (infectious mononucleosis)
		cytomegalovirus (CMV)	CMV retinitis (immunocompromised)
	Poxviridae	variola virus	smallpox
		vaccinia virus	vaccinia
single stranded DNA	Parvoviridae	human parvovirus B19	aplastic crisis in sickle cell disease patient

(table title: **Some important DNA viruses**)

RNA viruses

There are two types of ssRNA viruses, designated positive- and negative-sense viruses:

- In positive-sense viruses, the RNA can act as mRNA and is immediately translated into viral proteins.
- Negative-sense RNA cannot act as mRNA. Positive-sense RNA is synthesized from the negative strand with an RNA-dependent polymerase, which assembles from the nucleoprotein subunits in the viral particle when the virus first infects its host.

Examples of some important RNA viruses are given in Fig. 5.49.

Retroviruses (including HIV)

Retroviruses are positive-sense ssRNA viruses that produce a DNA intermediate with a unique enzyme called reverse transcriptase (Figs 5.50 and 5.51).

Human immunodeficiency viruses HIV-1 and HIV-2 are important retroviruses. They are responsible for the worldwide pandemic of acquired immunodeficiency syndrome (AIDS). HIV-1 has spread world wide; HIV-2 is localized to West Africa. In 1995, an estimated 18 million people were HIV positive. This is predicted to rise to 30–40 million by the year 2000.

HIV is transmitted:

- In blood (needlestick injury, sharing needles).

Fig. 5.49 Some important RNA viruses.

Some important RNA viruses			
Class	**Family**	**Species**	**Disease**
double stranded RNA	Reoviridae	human rotavirus	acute gastroenteritis
	Enteroviruses	poliovirus	polio
	Togaviridae	coxsackie B virus	myocarditis, aseptic meningitis
		echovirus	aseptic meningitis, exanthematous disease
	Orthomyxoviridae	rhinovirus	common cold
	Paramyxoviridae	hepatitis A	acute hepatitis
		yellow fever virus	yellow fever
		rubella virus	rubella (German measles)
		influenza A	influenza epidemics
		influenza B	influenza epidemics
		measles virus	measles
		mumps virus	mumps
positive-sense single stranded RNA	Arenaviridae	respiratory syncytial virus (RSV)	acute infantile bronchiolitis
		parainfluenza virus	croup
negative-sense single stranded RNA	Rhabdoviridae	lassa virus	lassa fever
		rabies virus	rabies

- By sexual contact (heterosexual and homosexual).
- From mother to baby.

HIV attacks the immune system and progressively destroys it. It specifically targets CD4-positive (CD4$^+$) cells (T helper cells and macrophages) by binding onto the CD4 receptor. The viral DNA integrates into the host genome and new virus particles are manufactured.

AIDS is characterized by features of severe immunodeficiency—severe and overwhelming infections and opportunistic cancers.

Drug treatment of HIV/AIDS

Current drug treatments aim to disable the HIV by inhibiting its enzymes. Combinations of drugs can greatly reduce virus load, but it has yet to be proved that they can eradicate the virus from a person who has HIV.

Zidovudine (also called azidothymidine, AZT) is a reverse transcriptase inhibitor. It is an analogue of thymidine that is phosphorylated in the host cell and competes with cellular triphosphates in the reverse transcription process. Host mitochondrial DNA polymerases are also susceptible to AZT and this probably brings about the side effects. These include anaemia and neutropenia, gastrointestinal disturbance, headache, fever, and skin rash.

Didanosine (ddI) is a synthetic purine dideoxynucleoside that works in the same way as AZT to inhibit reverse transcriptase. Protease inhibitors such as ritonavir target the enzyme that cuts up newly translated viral multiproteins into individual proteins to allow assembly of new viral particles.

Retroviruses do not possess a proofreader, so have a very high rate of uncorrected mutation: a new mutation occurs approximately every time the 9000 base pair genome is replicated. This leads to changes in the proteins of the viral coat and enzymes. Mutations tend to lead to resistance to drug treatments: for example, resistance to AZT developed over 12–18 months. Combinations of three drugs are therefore given to avoid the emergence of a resistant strain of the virus. Trials have shown that a combination of AZT, ddI, and a protease inhibitor can slow the disease progress.

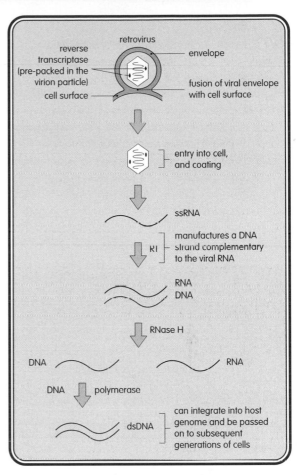

Fig. 5.50 Replication of retroviruses.

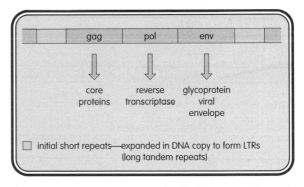

Fig. 5.51 Retrovirus genome—codes for three genes. These are preceded by a non-coding region containing enhancer and promoter regions which facilitate expression of the viral genome by host 'machinery'.

- ○ Describe the differences between bacterial and eukaryotic cells.
- ○ Explain the mechanisms of action of four types of antimicrobial agents. Give examples.
- ○ Describe how genetic material can be transferred between bacteria. Relate this to the development of antibiotic resistance.
- ○ Give examples of DNA viruses and explain the mechanism of replication.
- ○ Give examples of RNA viruses and explain the mechanism of replication.
- ○ Explain what is meant by a retrovirus, with the clinical example of HIV and AIDS.

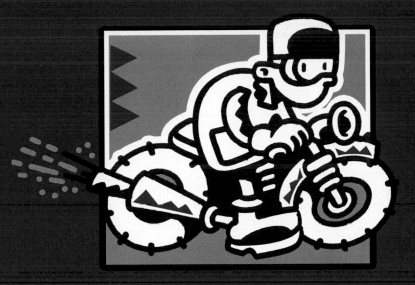

MEDICAL GENETICS

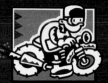

6. Principles of Medical Genetics

Genetic terminology used in inheritance

Genotype
This is the genetic constitution of an individual and is also used to refer to the alleles present at one locus.

Phenotype
This is the observed biochemical, physiological, or morphological characteristics of an individual that are determined by the genotype and the environment in which it is expressed.

Autosomes
These are any chromosomes other than sex chromosomes

Autosomal inheritance
This involves any chromosome other than the sex chromosomes.

Penetrance
Where a genetic lesion finds expression in some individuals, but not in others; penetrance is expressed as the proportion of individuals with the disease gene that have symptoms:
- If a genetic lesion is completely penetrant (100%) all the individuals with that altered gene express it (e.g. Huntington's chorea).
- About 75% of women with certain mutations in the BRCA1 gene develop breast or ovarian cancer (i.e. the mutations have a penetrance of 75%).

Variable expressivity
This occurs when a genetic lesion produces a range of phenotypes: for example, tuberous sclerosis can be asymptomatic with harmless kidney cysts, but in the next generation may be fatal, owing to the presence of brain malformations.

Heterozygote
This is an individual or genotype with two different alleles at a given locus on a pair of homologous chromosomes.

Homozygote
This is an individual or genotype with identical alleles at a given locus on a pair of homologous chromosomes.

Pedigree charts
These are used to illustrate inheritance (Fig. 6.1).

Mendelian inheritance
Mendelian inheritance follows specific patterns, which determine risk to relatives. Single gene disorders, which are due to one or more mutant alleles at a single locus, follow simple mendelian inheritance.

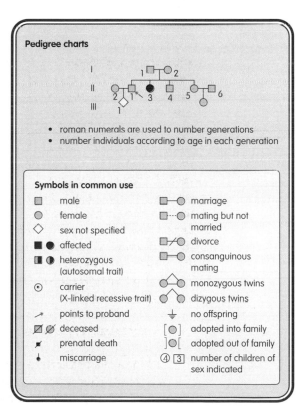

Fig. 6.1 Symbols and configuration of pedigree charts.

Autosomal dominant (AD)

A dominant gene is phenotypically expressed in homozygotes and heterozygotes for that gene (Fig. 6.2). In this pattern of inheritance:

- There is vertical inheritance (affected parent has an affected child).
- Unaffected family members usually have unaffected partners and produce normal children.
- Affected family members usually have unaffected partners and produce a 1:1 ratio of normal and affected children.
- Usually both sexes are equally affected and they are equally likely to pass on the disease.
- Common autosomal dominant diseases are achondroplasia, Huntington's disease, retinoblastoma and neurofibromatosis type I.

Homozygotes for the trait are rare. In some AD conditions, new mutations account for a substantial proportion of cases (e.g. achondroplasia, familial adenomatous polyposis). AD genes can show:

- Sex limitation (e.g. balding, gout, male-limited precocious puberty, familial breast/ovarian cancer).
- Reduced penetrance (e.g. retinoblastoma).
- Variable expressivity (e.g. tuberous sclerosis).
- Imprinting (see p. 108).
- Anticipation (see p. 107).

Autosomal recessive (AR)

A recessive gene or trait is expressed only in homozygotes for the abnormal gene (Fig. 6.3). In autosomal recessive inheritance:

- There is horizontal inheritance (normal parents often have more than one affected child).
- Affected individuals have phenotypically normal parents.
- Affected individuals usually have unaffected partners and all their children will be carriers.
- If a carrier has an unaffected partner, there is a 50% chance of the children being carriers.
- Only matings between heterozygotes will produce affected individuals, with an expectation of 1 in 4.
- There is an association with consanguinity due to sharing of genes in families (more likely if the gene is rare).
- Both sexes are equally affected.
- Common diseases are cystic fibrosis, Tay–Sachs disease, phenylketonuria (PKU).

Consanguinity is where there is a mating between two people who have a familial relationship closer than that of second cousins.

AR genes may show a sex influence: for example, haemochromatosis is autosomal recessive but has a

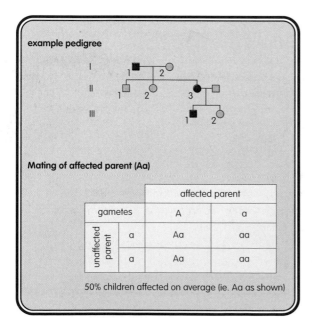

example pedigree

Mating of affected parent (Aa)

gametes	affected parent	
	A	a
unaffected parent — a	Aa	aa
unaffected parent — a	Aa	aa

50% children affected on average (ie. Aa as shown)

Fig. 6.2 Example pedigree and typical offspring of mating in AD inheritance. (A, disease allele.)

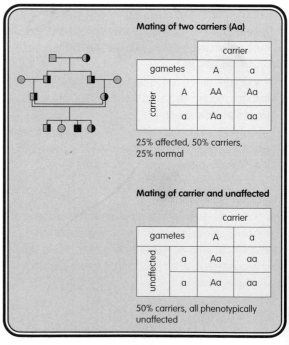

Mating of two carriers (Aa)

gametes	carrier	
	A	a
carrier — A	AA	Aa
carrier — a	Aa	aa

25% affected, 50% carriers, 25% normal

Mating of carrier and unaffected

gametes	carrier	
	A	a
unaffected — a	Aa	aa
unaffected — a	Aa	aa

50% carriers, all phenotypically unaffected

Fig. 6.3 Example pedigree and typical offspring of matings in AR inheritance. (A, disease allele.)

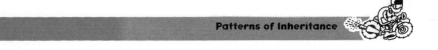

higher incidence in males due to lower dietary iron intake and menstruation in females.

Autosomal codominant

Both alleles, A and a, are expressed in the heterozygote, giving a different phenotype from authosomal recessive and aa. The inheritance is similar to autosomal recessive. Many biochemical variants are codominant, for example:

- ABO blood group.
- Haemoglobin S (heterozygote has sickling trait, homozygote has sickling disease).

Sex-linked

Genes located on the X chromosome are said to be X-linked, whereas genes on the Y chromosome are said to be Y-linked. Males are hemizygous (only have one chromosome) for the X chromosome. For X-linked recessive genes the inheritance pattern (Fig. 6.4) is as follows:

- More males than females show the recessive phenotype.
- The disease is transmitted by a carrier female, who is usually asymptomatic.
- If a mother is a carrier her sons have a 50% chance of being affected and her daughters a 50% chance of being carriers.

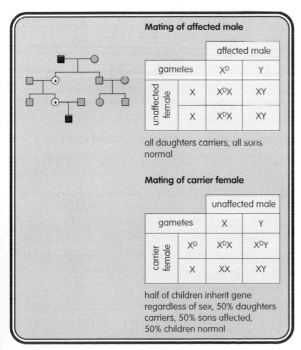

Fig. 6.4 Example pedigree and typical offspring of mating in X-linked recessive inheritance. (D, disease allele.)

- An affected male will usually have no affected offspring, but all the daughters will be carriers and, in turn, 50% of their sons will be affected.
- No sons of the affected male will inherit the gene (i.e. there is no male-to-male transmission).
- Affected males may have unaffected parents but will often have an affected maternal uncle or cousin.

Common X-linked recessive diseases are Duchenne muscular dystrophy and haemophilia A.

About 35% of mutations in lethal X-linked recessive conditions are new. Women can be affected with X-linked recessive conditions if an affected male mates with a carrier female, if there is lyonization (inactivation) of a normal X chromosome in a skewed pattern, if there is X chromosome autosome translocation, or if XO (Turner's syndrome) is present.

The X-linked dominant inheritance pattern is rare and difficult to distinguish from AD except that affected males have normal sons, but all daughters are affected, for example Xg blood group, X-linked hypophosphataemic rickets, Rett syndrome (X-linked dominant and only seen in females as lethal in males).

Y-linked (holandric) inheritance is very rare (e.g. hairy ears).

Non-mendelian inheritance

Penetrance and expressivity

A full explanation of penetrance and expressivity is given on p. 111.

Anticipation

This is where certain mendelian genes will manifest a phenotype with decreased age of onset and often of increased severity as they are inherited through generations. The mutations in these genes are due to trinucleotide repeat expansions (e.g. Huntington's chorea, Myotonic Dystrophy).

Mosaicism

A mosaic is an individual with multiple cell lines (genotypes) from a single zygote. Mosaicism can be an important clinical factor in:

- Cancers caused by somatic mutations generating genetically distinct sublines.
- Some instances of chromosomal disorders (e.g. mild cases of Down syndrome may occur due to the formation of a trisomy cell line (46 XX or 47 XY + 21) during the early stages of division of a normal (46 XX or XY) zygote.

Germline mosaicism occurs when an abnormal cell line is confined to the gonads, and may account for apparently unaffected parents producing more than one child with an AD condition.

Somatic mosaicism is where either the paternal or maternal representative of a chromosome is randomly inactivated in each somatic cell and, once established, will be inactivated in all daughter cells. It may account for:

- Unusually mild symptoms in AD metabolic conditions if there is disproportional inactivation of the aberrant gene.
- Expression of X-linked disease alleles in female carriers if there is disproportionate inactivation of the normal gene.

Imprinting

This is differential expression of genetic material at chromosomal or allelic level, depending upon which parent (male or female) it has been inherited from. It can be thought of as selective inactivation of genes (probably through methylation) according to the paternal or maternal origins of the chromosomes. Hydatidiform moles illustrate the different roles of paternal and maternal genomes:

- A complete mole (46 XX) has chromosomes that are all paternal in origin (both X chromosomes being of paternal origin, ie extra paternal set, but no maternal set), and results in either no fetus or a normal placenta with severe hyperplasia of the cytotrophoblast.
- A partial mole (69) is a triploid with an extra set of chromosomes of maternal or paternal origin. An extra paternal set (diandric) results in abundant trophoblast, but poor embryonic development. An extra maternal set (digynic) results in severely retarded embryonic development with a small fibrotic placenta.

Prader–Willi and Angelman syndromes

The microdeletion syndromes Prader–Willi and Angelman syndromes are phenotypically distinct because of imprinting. In both there is an identical microdeletion of chromosome 15 (q11–13) with the phenotype being due to differential parental inactivation of the residual non-deleted copy:

- Prader–Willi syndrome is due to paternal deletion, so will have only the maternal contribution, where the PW gene is switched off.
- Angelman syndrome is due to maternal deletion, so will have only the paternal contribution, (Fig. 6.5) where the AS gene is switched off.

Uniparental disomy

This is caused by duplication of a chromosome from one parent with loss of the corresponding homologue from the other parent (Fig. 6.6): for example, uniparental disomy of maternal chromosome 15 can result in the same phenotype as Prader–Willi, but with no deletion as there will be no paternal contribution to chromosome 15. A few cases of cystic fibrosis with severe growth retardation have two homologous chromosomes 7 of maternal origin, and probably growth retardation reflects imprinting of a growth function gene. Beckwith–Wiedemann syndrome can be due to paternal duplication of 11p15.

Mitochondrial inheritance

Mitochondria have their own DNA and are inherited only from the mother, as ova have an abundant cytoplasm containing mitochondria; the sperm contributes no mitochondria to the zygote.

Mitochondria are distributed randomly in daughter cells, so these may contain normal mitochondrial DNA, mutant DNA, or a mixture of both. There is, therefore, variable expression of disease due to mutation in mitochondrial DNA, depending upon the relative

| paternal derived Ch15 imprinting—inactivates Angelman's syndrome gene (AS) | maternal derived Ch15 imprinting—inactivates Prader–Willi syndrome gene (PW) |

PW gene

off ⌐ AS gene

off ⌐ PW gene

AS gene

Paternal Ch missing—Prader–Willi syndrome due to lack of PW gene

Maternal Ch missing—Angelman syndrome due to lack of AS gene

Fig. 6.5 How deletion of one parental chromosome 15 with imprinting of the present chromosome 15 can lead to Prader–Willi or Angelman syndrome. Normal development requires both maternal and paternally derived genes to be expressed.

proportion of normal to mutant DNA. No affected male will transmit the disease (e.g. Leber's optic atrophy).

Polygenic and multifactorial inheritance
Polygenic inheritance
In polygenic inheritance, a number of genes operate together quantitatively to determine a particular characteristic (e.g. intelligence, height). In multifactorial inheritance, a trait is determined by a combination of both genes and environmental factors and can be classified as:

- Congenital malformations—for example, neural tube defects, congenital dislocation of the hip (CDH), pyloric stenosis, cleft lip and palate, congenital heart disease.
- Common disorders of adult life—for example, diabetes mellitus, peptic ulcers, coronary artery disease, schizophrenia.

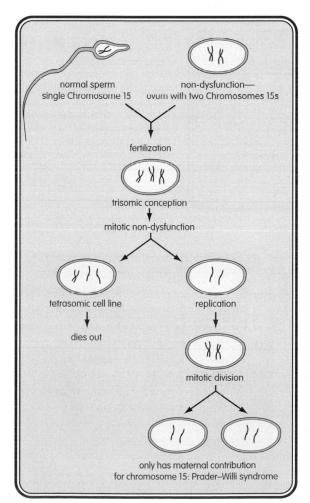

Fig. 6.6 Mechanism of uniparental disomy (here for chromosome 15).

- Normal human characteristics—for example, blood pressure, height, finger ridges, intelligence.

A continuous (Gaussian) normal distribution curve is typical, but not diagnostic, of multifactorial inheritance (i.e. abnormalities do not usually have a distinct phenotype but are extremes of the curve, with exceptions having distinct phenotypes, e.g. peptic ulcer). The number of genes involved may be very few as, even when a single locus is implicated, variation in the environment can ensure normal distribution of the trait.

Twin studies show the importance of genes and the environment. For example, cleft lip and palate has a population incidence of 1 in 1000, but:

- Concordance in monozygotic twins is 40% (if due only to genes there would be 100% concordance, so genes are important but other factors are also involved).
- Concordance in dizygotic twins is 4% (these twins have different genes but the same environment, showing the importance of environmental factors).

CDH is an example of multifactorial inheritance:

- The genetic factors are acetabular dysplasia, familial general joint laxity, and transient joint laxity at pregnancy term.
- The environmental factors are position of the legs *in utero* and after birth.

Threshold model of multifactorial inheritance
Fig. 6.7 shows the threshold model of multifactorial inheritance. Distribution of risk genes in the population is normal. An individual's risk genes and environmental predisposition are collectively termed the individual's liability. If the liability is above the genetic threshold, the

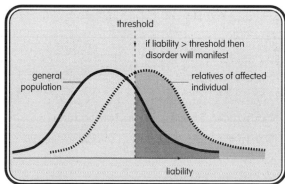

Fig. 6.7 Threshold model of multifactorial inheritance.

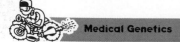

disorder will manifest. The proportion greater than the threshold is equal to the population incidence. The liability curve is shifted to the right for relatives of an affected individual.

Heritability

This refers to how much of a disease can be ascribed to genetic rather than environmental factors and is expressed as a percentage, with higher values when the genetic contribution is more important (e.g. heritability of schizophrenia is 85% and that of peptic ulcer is 37%).

If heritability is high, there is a high correlation in relatives (e.g. finger ridge correlation in first degree relatives is 0.49). Usually heritability is low, so the incidence in relatives falls off sharply (e.g. cleft lip and palate, Fig. 6.8). Empirical risks, calculated from relatives,

are used in genetic counselling as there is no predictable pattern of inheritance.

Risk rates of recurrence depend upon:
- Severity of the disorder in the affected person (e.g. severe bilateral cleft lip is more likely to recur in siblings than unilateral cleft lip).
- Number of affected individuals in a family.
- Sex affected.

There is a sex difference in population incidence: for example, pyloric stenosis is more common in boys, so children of an affected female will be more likely to develop the condition than children of an affected male, as the female needs a high number of risk genes to manifest the condition.

Fig. 6.9 lists the differences between mendelian and multifactorial inheritance.

Risk to relatives for multifactorial disorders				
Disorder	Relative risk disorder			
	1° relative	2° relative	3° relative	General population
Cleft lip and palate	4	0.6	0.3	0.1
Neural tube defects	4	1.5	0.6	0.3
Epilepsy	5	2.5	1.5	1.0

Fig. 6.8 Risk to relatives for multifactorial disorders. First degree relatives are parents, siblings and offspring (share 50% of genome); second degree relatives are grandparents, aunts and uncles, grandchildren (share 25% of genome); third degree relatives include cousins and great-grandchildren (share 12.5% of genome).

Differences between mendelian and multifactorial inheritance	
Mendelian	Multifactorial
all or nothing	additive with a varying phenotype
If you have the gene, you have the disease	possible to have lots of contributing genes, but if less than the threshold, do not have the disease
risk does not increase through life	can acquire more liability through life

Fig. 6.9 Differences between mendelian and multifactorial inheritance.

- Construct pedigree charts using the standard symbols.
- Describe the patterns of mendelian inheritance, with examples.
- Define anticipation, mosaicism, imprinting, uniparental disomy, and mitochondrial inheritance.
- Discuss the difference between polygenic and multifactorial inheritance.
- Discuss the threshold model.

GENETICS IN DISEASE

Chromosomal disorders

Chromosomal disorders occur in over 7.5% of conceptions, but live birth incidence is only 6/1000 since most end in spontaneous abortion. Chromosomal disorders may be numerical or structural. Numerical disorders may result from:

- Extra single chromosomes (e.g. trisomy).
- Missing single chromosomes (e.g. monosomy—lethal except for XO).
- Extra haploid sets (e.g. tetraploids or triploids).

Aneuploidy means any chromosome number that is not an exact multiple of the haploid number, for example:

- Trisomy 21 (Down syndrome).
- Monosomy X (Turner's syndrome).

Aneuploids arise by non-disjunction or chromosome lag at meiosis or mitosis. Fig. 6.10 shows the mechanisms of non-dysjunction and chromosome lag.
Polyploidy means an abnormal chromosomal complement that exceeds the diploid number and is an exact multiple of the haploid number. Polyploids arise from fertilization by two sperm, failed first zygotic division, or failed maturation division.

Structural disorders include translocation, inversion, isochromosome, duplication, deletion, and ring chromosomes. All structural disorders result from breakage (Fig. 6.11). Chromosomal damage is increased by:

- Some environmental conditions (e.g. mutagenic chemicals, radiation).
- Genetic chromosome instability disorders (e.g. ataxia telangiectasia and Fanconi's syndrome).

Translocation

This is the (usually reciprocal) exchange of chromosome segments that usually involves dissimilar chromosomes (Figs 6.12 and 6.13). In translocations there is usually no loss of genetic material, so there is a normal phenotype, called a balanced carrier. Prenatal diagnosis may be carried out for balanced carriers as the gametes may be unbalanced.

Inversion

This arises when two breaks occur in the chromosome and the intervening DNA rotates through 180 degrees. Paracentric inversions occur if the breaks occur in one arm, whereas pericentric inversions involve the centromere (Figs 6.14 and 6.15). In meiosis, homologous chromosomes can pair only if a loop is formed in the region of the inversion. Paracentric gametes are non-viable, whereas pericentric gametes are usually viable.

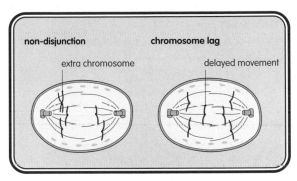

Fig. 6.10 Mechanisms of non-disjunction and chromosome lag. In non-disjunction there is failed separation of paired chromosomes, or sister chromatids separate at anaphase. The chromosome lag shows the delayed movement of a chromosome at anaphase (which usually affects only one of the daughter cells).

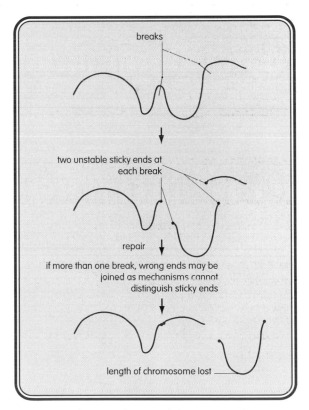

Fig. 6.11 Mechanism of structural chromosome damage, due to the limitations of DNA repair systems.

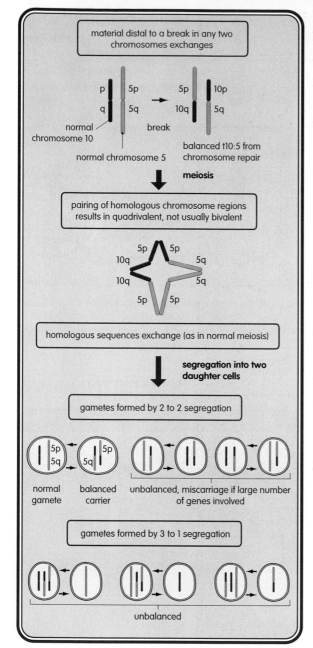

Fig. 6.12 Mechanism of reciprocal translocation (highly simplified).

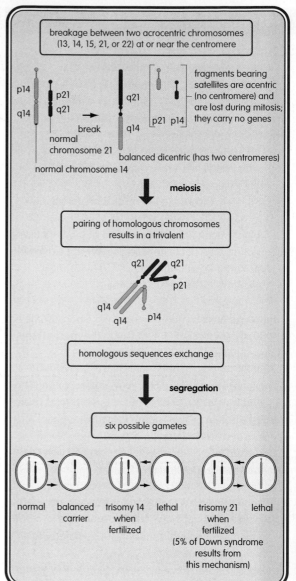

Fig. 6.13 Mechanism of Robertsonian (centric) translocation (highly simplified).

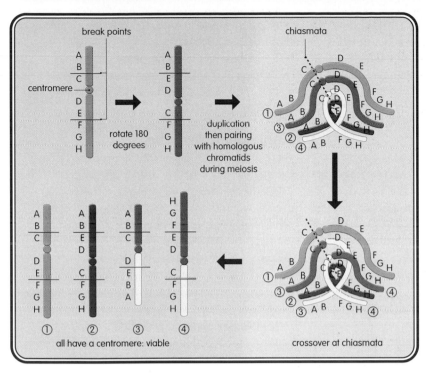

Fig. 6.14 Mechanism of pericentric inversion.

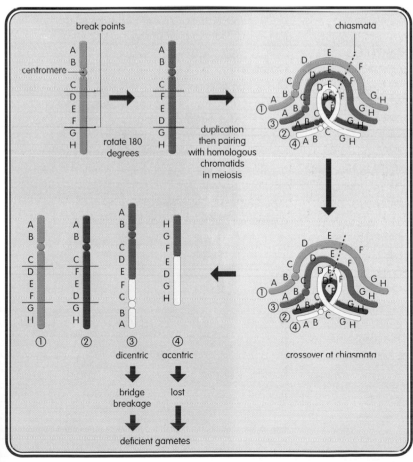

Fig. 6.15 Mechanism of paracentric inversion.

Isochromosome

This chromosome has a duplication of one arm, but lacks the other. It results from breakage of a chromatid with fusion above the centromere or transverse division. It occurs in 17% of cases of Turner's syndrome.

Duplication

This implies an extra copy of a chromosome region. Causes include inheritance from parents with balanced structural disorders and *de novo* duplication from unequal crossing-over in meiosis, translocation, or inversion.

Deletion and ring chromosome

Deletion results in a loss of genetic material. The telomere is important in chromosome function, so interstitial deletions are more common. If a deleted fragment has no centromere it will be lost during mitosis.

Ring chromosomes result from breaks near both telomeres of a chromosome, which aberrantly repair to form a ring, with the regions distal to the breaks being lost. If the ring has a centromere it will be passed through generations.

Visible structural deletions are large, with the smallest being at least 3 million base pairs (Mbp) (microdeletions). Single gene disorders may be caused by deletions, but if the deletions are not visible by light microscopy they are not considered structural. Structural deletions may cause deletion syndromes with more than one single gene disorder occurring concurrently.

All chromosomal disorders are individually rare, with no clear patterns of inheritance and minimal risk to relatives. International Standard Chromosome Nomenclature (ISCN) is as follows:

- Numerical disorders are described as follows—number of chromosomes, sex chromosomes, + or − chromosome number, for example, boy with trisomy 21 is [47, XY, + 21], Turner's syndrome is [45, X].
- Structural disorders are described as follows—number of chromosomes, sex chromosomes, mutation (chromosomes involved), (break points, margins or region) (p, short arm; q, long arm).

Examples of ISCN for structural disorders include the following:

- Translocation (t)—[46, XY, t(14;21) (q11;p10)].
- Inversion (inv)—[46, XY, inv(9)(p12,q14)] pericentric inversion.

- Isochromosome (I) —[46, X, I(Xq)] long chromosome arm of X duplicated.
- Duplication (dup)—[46, XY, dup(5)(q20–q30)].
- Deletion (del) and ring chromosome (r)—[46 XY, del(15)(q11–q13)] in Prader–Willi syndrome; [46 XX, r(X)(p12,q14)].

Single gene disorders

There are approximately 6000 single gene disorders. Individually they are rare, usually affecting from 1 in 10 000, to 1 in 100 000. AD incidence is 2–9 in 1000 people. AR incidence is 2 in 1000 people. Most AR conditions have a carrier frequency of 1 in 100 unless unusually common (e.g. cystic fibrosis). X-linked recessive incidence is 0.5–2 in 1000 males. Cumulatively, single gene disorders are common, affecting 1% of the population. They follow mendelian inheritance patterns, so imply high risk to relatives.

Mutations in single gene disorders arise from deletion, insertion, duplication, inversions, or point mutations. Mutations are random inheritable changes in the amount or structure of genetic material that can be inherited or arise spontaneously. Hugo DeVries introduced the mutation concept in 1901.

Deletion

This is loss of chromosomal material involving from one to many thousands of base pairs. Deletions result from unequal crossing-over, chromosome breakage, and structural disorders. Sequences at the end of deletions are often similar, as these predispose to slippage during replication, hence recombination errors (Fig. 6.16). Runs of bases and repeated motifs also predispose to deletion by replication slippage.

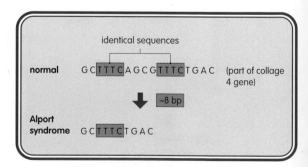

Fig. 6.16 Deletion in Alport's syndrome. (A, adenine; bp, base pairs; C, cytosine, G, guanine, T, thymine. Part of collage 4 gene.)

Insertion

This is gain in chromosomal material involving from just one to many thousands of base pairs. Duplication is a special type of insertion that is identical to an adjacent sequence. Runs of bases and repeated motifs predispose to duplication by replication slippage (Fig. 6.17). Triplet repeats are duplications.

Inversion

These involve from just two to many thousands of base pairs. Sequences at the ends often resemble each other. In haemophilia A, 40% of mutations result from an inversion of several hundred thousand base pairs within the factor VIII gene.

Point mutation

This is a single base substitution with no net gain or loss of chromosomal material. Substitutions are classified as:

- Transition—purine to purine or pyrimidine to pyrimidine.
- Transversion—purine to pyrimidine or vice versa.

Point mutations may be silent, deleterious, or advantageous. Deleterious substitution effect depends upon the site:

- In the gene codon they are silent if the new triplet codes the same amino acid, missense if it codes a different amino acid, and nonsense if it codes a stop codon.
- In the splice site or regulatory region they produce qualitative and quantitative effects, respectively.

Deletions and insertions may affect anything from one exon to many genes. The effect depends upon the amount of material lost or gained and whether the reading frame is affected. The transcript is read in triplet codons. If a small insertion or deletion mutation is divisible by three, there is a change in the number of amino acids in the protein product. If not divisible by three, the reading frame will be shifted and result in truncation of the protein, because misreading of the codons beyond the frameshift will inevitably generate a 'stop' signal.

Diseases may be caused by one type of mutation or many mutations (heterogeneous). The factors affecting mutation type and frequency are:

- Natural selection—harmful genes would normally be removed from the gene pool over many generations. Sickle cell heterozygotes are less susceptible to malaria, so selective advantage maintains gene frequency.
- Drift—this is a change in allele proportions in the population by random events. Small populations can have a large standard error, so drift can be profound (called the founder effect). Disease genes that originate from a small population, appear through consanguinity if autosomal recessive; this is less common today (e.g. 78% of cases of cystic fibrosis are due to the deletion F508, even though over 400 other mutations have been identified).
- Mutation frequency—the dystrophin gene lies close to a recombination hot spot resulting in a large number of deletions. Factor VIII contains a repeat sequence that predisposes to inversion mutations. Increasing paternal age increases the chance of AD mutation (e.g. achondroplasia).
- Migration—this allows gene flow, so new alleles may be introduced (e.g. increased blood group B in UK population due to Asian immigration).
- Non-random mating—consanguinity increases the chance of a homozygous recessive condition. The rarer the AR condition, the greater the chance that an affected individual is the product of consanguineous mating.
- Sensitivity to subtle changes—the factor VIII gene is susceptible to minor mutations as the nature of each amino acid sequence is critical to function, so these are often found. The dystrophin gene is tolerant to minor changes, so, large mutations are found in the disease gene.

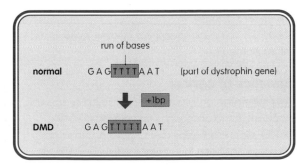

Fig. 6.17 Duplication in Duchenne muscular dystrophy (DMD). (A, adenine; bp, base pairs; C, cytosine, G, guanine, T, thymine.)

In many cases the severity of the disease may be related to the mutation type.

Trinucleotide repeat disorders

These disorders result from expansion of a contiguous triplet nucleotide repeat within, or very close to, the gene. For example:

- Fragile chromosome site mental retardation syndromes (e.g. fragile X syndrome).
- Neurodegenerative disorders such as Huntington's disease.
- Myotonic dystrophy.

All these repeats involve cytosine/guanine (C/G)-rich trinucleotides (CGG, CCG, CAG, CTG), and may involve a few copies to several thousand repeats. Anticipation is seen in many of these disorders. For definition of anticiption see p. 113.

- Huntington's disease repeat lengths: normal individuals have 6 to 37 trinucleotide repeats, whereas Huntington's disease patients have 30 to 121 repeats

There is an overlap in the number of repeats seen in normal and diseased phenotypes, but vast majority of Huntington's disease alleles and normal alleles are well within their respective ranges.

There is an inverse correlation between repeat length and age of onset. This is marked in juvenile cases, but adult onset is variable and age is only weakly related to repeat length. As the repeat increases it becomes less stable during replication. Repeat instability in somatic cells or between generations is the cause for acceleration of gene expansion. Studies show that normal alleles have repeat stability, thus the initial origin of expansions is unknown. Intergenerational repeat instability of disease alleles may show sex bias: e.g. maternal transmission of Huntington's disease repeat shows small (less than five repeats) increases or decreases, whereas paternal transmission of Huntington's disease shows small (less than five repeats) or large (up to 74 repeats) increases.

Polygenic inheritance of common diseases

Individual disorders are common, affecting 2–3 in 1000 people. Heritability is the proportion of a trait that can be attributed to genetic factors. The numbers of genes involved are unknown for each disease, but a normal distribution curve can be achieved with only a few loci. Genes that are associated with a disease may not cause that disease, but may be associated, owing to linkage disequilibrium.

Genetic factors contributing to common polygenic diseases

Diabetes mellitus (insulin dependent)

There is 40% concordance in monozygotic twins: 98% are major histocompatibility complex (MHC) DR3 or DR4 and B8. Only 50% of non-diabetics have these MHC alleles. Aspartate at the DQ locus is protective—19% of the general population and 95% of the IDDM population are aspartate negative. Other loci involved are on 14q and 11p.

Essential hypertension

The heritability of essential hypertension is 62%. Genes are important in causing hypertension and the response to treatment.

Atherosclerosis

The heritability is about 65%. Heritable factors are hypertension, diabetes mellitus, premature ischaemic heart disease, and abnormal lipoprotein profiles—elevated low-density lipoprotein (LDL) and high-density lipoprotein (HDL).

Lipoprotein profile has been associated with single gene disorders and the polygenic inheritance of some genes such as *Apo* AI and *Apo* CIII. (Apo, apolipoprotein)

Peptic ulcer

The heritability is 37%, and 50% of affected families have increased pepsinogen I, which is inherited as AD.

Schizophrenia

The heritability is 85%. It may be associated with a locus on 5q, though in some studies this is controversial.

Asthma

The heritability is 80% and is associated with HLA A23.

Alzheimer's disease

About 10% of patients inherit this disease as AD linked to chromosome 21.

Genetics of cancer

Cell proliferation and survival are controlled by growth-promoting proto-oncogenes and growth-inhibiting tumour suppressor gene (see Chapter 5). No single oncogene has been found that is altered in 100% of tumours. Fig. 6.18 shows the pathway to malignancy.

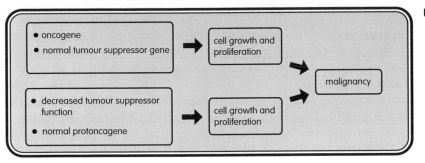

Fig. 6.18 Pathway to malignancy.

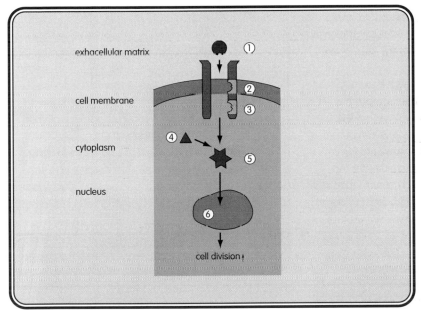

Fig. 6.19 Classes of oncogene by transduction position. (1) Growth factors (e.g. platelet-derived growth factor (PPGF) *sis*. (2) Growth factor receptors (e.g. EGFR—*Gb*. (3) Post-receptor proteins (e.g. *ras*). (4) Postreceptor tyrosine kinase (e.g. *abl, src*). (5) Cytoplasmic proteins (e.g. raf). (6) Nuclear proteins (e.g. *myc*).

Fig. 6.20 Categories of oncogenes.

Categories of oncogenes			
	Function	**Mutation**	**Examples**
Category I (growth and proliferation genes)	I. transcription factors	gain of function	*myc*
	II. cyclins		*abl*
	III. mediate signal transduction		*ras, bcl-1*
Category II (tumour suppressor genes)	I. inhibit growth and proliferation	loss of function	*Rb, p53*
Category III (programmed cell death genes)	I. abrogate cell death	gain of function	*bcl-2*
	II. promote cell death	loss of function	*p53*

Oncogenes

Proto-oncogenes are normal genes that tend to promote normal cell growth. Oncogene activation from proto-oncogenes leads to abnormal cell control. Oncogenes can be classified by transduction position or functional category (Fig. 6.19). Fig. 6.20 describes the different categories of oncogenes.

Activation of oncogenes occurs by:

- Translocation (e.g. Burkitt's lymphoma (t8;14) or t(8;2) activates c-*myc* on 8q.
- Amplification, (e.g. n-*myc* amplified in neuroblastoma).
- Point mutation in oncogene (e.g. Ha-*ras* mutation in bladder cancer).

Tumour suppressor genes

These are also known as anti-oncogenes and they normally inhibit tumorigenesis (Figs 6.21 and 6.22). Tumours develop if there is loss of both wild-type alleles. The heterozygote form predisposes to cancer.

Tumour suppressor genes are vulnerable sites for critical DNA damage since loss of function contributes to tumorigenesis. Loss of activity can be through damage to

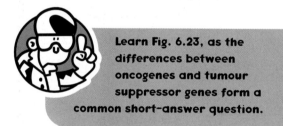

Learn Fig. 6.23, as the differences between oncogenes and tumour suppressor genes form a common short-answer question.

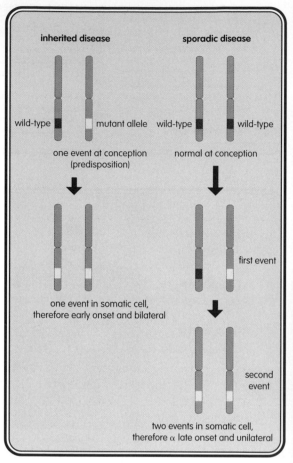

Fig. 6.21 Knudson 'two-hit' hypothesis. Note that two events must occur to lose tumour repressor function.

Fig. 6.22 Examples of tumour suppressor genes.

Tumour suppressor genes			
Gene	**Locus**	**Function**	**Tumour**
Rb	13q14	substrate of CDK (cell cycle regulation)	retinoblastoma, osteosarcoma
p53	17p13	growth arrest and apoptosis	mutated in 70% of all human tumours
WT-1	11p13	zinc finger	Wilms' tumour
NF-1	17q	transcription factor	neurofibromatosis
APC	5q21	cell adhesion	adenomatous polyposis
DCC	18q21	cell adhesion	colorectal cancer, pancreatic cancer, oesophageal cancer

Differences between oncogenes and tumour suppressor genes	
Oncogene	**Tumour suppressor gene**
gene active in tumour	gene inactive in tumour
specific translocations/point mutations	deletions or mutations
mutations rarely hereditary	mutations can be inherited
dominant at cell level	recessive at cell level
broad tissue specificity	considerable tumour specificity
especially leukaemia and lymphoma	solid tumours

Fig. 6.23 Differences between oncogenes and tumour suppressor genes.

the genome (e.g. mutation, rearrangement, non-disjunction, gene conversion, imprinting, mitotic recombination), or interaction with cellular or viral proteins (e.g. MDM2, HPV E6 antigen, adenovirus E1b protein).

Tumour suppressor genes are important in:
- Inherited predisposition to cancer.
- Early events in tumorigenesis (they cooperate with dominant transforming genes to cause neoplasia).
- Disease markers ((e.g. presymptomatic diagnosis of adenomatous polyposis coli by demonstrating *APC* (adenomatous polyposis coli) gene mutation).

Tumour suppressor genes are potential targets for gene therapy (see pp. 141–142).

Multistage process of carcinogenesis
Carcinogenesis requires the accumulation of many mutant genes. It can be thought of as tumour evolution with each mutation acquisition forming a new clone (Fig. 6.24).

Familial cancer syndromes
These mendelian traits are:
- AD cancer traits (e.g. multiple endocrine neoplasia types 1 and 2, adenomatous polyposis coli, familial breast/ovarian cancer).
- DNA repair defects and chromosome instability (e.g. ataxia telangiectasia, Fanconi's anaemia).
- Hamartomatous syndromes (e.g. tuberous sclerosis, Cowden's disease) (see p. 168).

Features that suggest predisposition are:
- Family history of the same cancer, an associated cancer, or a rare cancer (e.g. retinoblastoma).

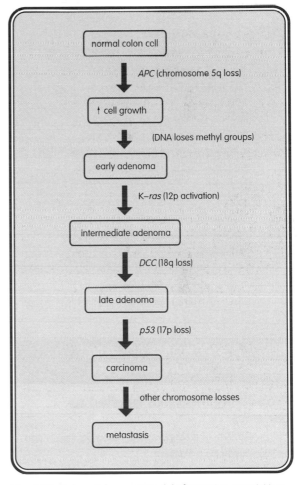

Fig. 6.24 Colorectal cancer model of mutation acquisition.

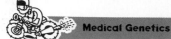

- Diagnosis at an early age (e.g. colon cancer in 20s in adenomatous polyposis coli).
- Multifocal or bilateral neoplasia including multiple cancers in associated sites (e.g. bilateral breast and ovarian cancer).
- Features that suggest a mendelian cancer—predisposing condition (e.g. skin hamartomas and enlarged cranium in Cowden's disease).

- **Name and describe the varieties of numerical disorders.**
- **Define the mechanisms of structural disorders by translocation, inversion, isochromosome, duplication, deletion, and ring chromosome.**
- **Define the mutations causing single gene disorders and their possible effect on the reading frame.**
- **Name examples of genetic factors in polygenic disorders.**
- **Describe the multistage process of carcinogenesis.**

RISK ASSESSMENT AND GENETIC COUNSELLING

Probability theory as applied to genetics

The probability of a single event occurring event can be expressed as a fraction:

$$p = \frac{\text{number of ways events can happen}}{\text{total number of possibilities}}$$

Probability is a useful way of demonstrating the risk of specific genetic event(s) occurring.

Laws of addition and multiplication of probability

If two events could not happen at the same time, they are said to be mutually exclusive. The probability that either event will occur is equal to the sum of their probabilities. The law of addition is:

$$P = p_1 + p_2$$

An independent event is one that has no effect on subsequent events. The outcome of the first event has no effect on subsequent events. The probability that all the events will occur is equal to the product of the individual probabilities. The law of multiplication is:

$$P = p_1 \times p_2$$

The law of multiplication is sometimes called the 'and' law because it is the probability that one event 'and' another event will occur.

Bayes' theorem

This is the method of determining the relative probabilities of two alternative outcomes:
- The 'prior' probability is based on classical Mendelian inheritance
- The 'conditional' probability is based on observations that modify the prior probability, such as existing unaffected offspring and results of screening tests.

A 'joint' probability is the calculated as the product the prior and the conditional probability. A final 'relative' probability is the proportional risk of the one alternative with respect to the other.

Calculating risks

Figs 6.27–6.29 provide examples of how common genetic risks can be calculated.

Aspects of genetic counselling
Establishing the diagnosis

Genetic counselling (see Chapter 7) is the provision of information to affected individuals or family members at risk of a disorder that may be genetic. The consultands (individuals attending counselling) are informed of:
- The consequences of the disorder.
- The probability of developing or transmitting it.
- Ways in which it may be prevented or ameliorated.

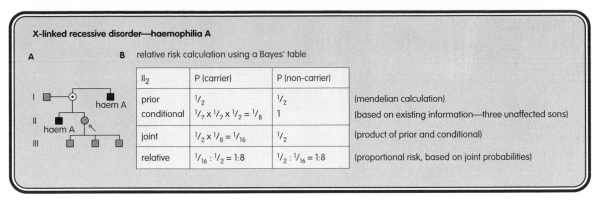

Fig. 6.25 Estimation of carrier risk using Bayes' theorem. (A) Mother (I₂) is an obligate carrier as she has an affected brother and son. Daughter (II₂) has already had three unaffected sons. What is the risk that she is affected? (B) The relative risk calculated can be displayed on a Bayes' table.

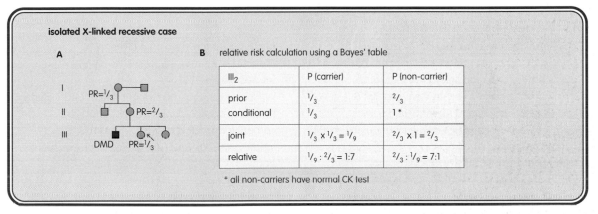

Fig. 6.26 Estimation of carrier risk using Bayes' theorem II. (A) Isolated case of DMD in III₁; assess carrier risk in his sister, III₂. 35% of cases arise from new mutations — neither mother nor sister would undergo mutation. If mutation was inherited from the mother, the carrier risk for the sister would be halved. If the mutation was from the grandmother, the mother would be an obligate carrier (carrier risk) 1 and the daughter's carrier risk would be half. Based on this information, prior risk for the grandmother is one-third, the mother is two-thirds, and the daughter is one-third. The daughter has a normal creatine kinase (CK) test. In general, two-thirds of carriers have raised CK and one-third have normal CK. (B) The relative risk calculated can be displayed on a Bayes' table.

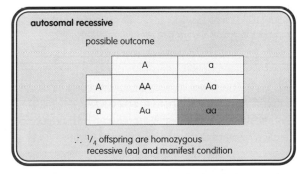

Fig. 6.27 Mendelian inheritance and risk calculation I. The condition manifests itself only when it is homozygous. If both parents are carriers of the allele, the risk of developing the condition is one-quarter. (a, mutant allele; A, normal allele.)

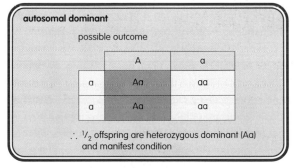

Fig. 6.28 Mendelian inheritance and risk calculation II. Only one copy of mutant allele is needed to manifest symptoms. If one parent is affected, the risk of having an affected child is one-half. (a, recessive non-mutant allele; A, dominant mutant allele.)

127

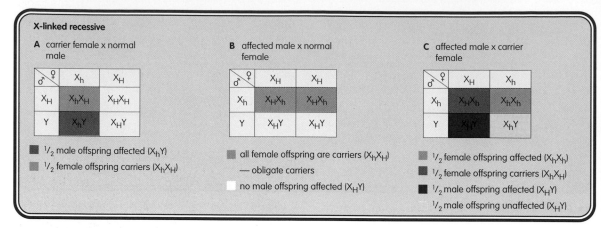

Fig. 6.29 Mendelian inheritance and risk calculation III. The mutant allele is expressed in all males since only one copy of X-linked alleles carried. Affected male passes allele on to all female offspring and no male offspring, e.g. haemophilia A. (X_h, mutant allele; X_H, normal allele.)

An accurate diagnosis is essential to genetic counselling so that the correct advice can be given. A medical history of all affected family individuals is needed and a pedigree constructed (see Fig. 6.1). Miscarriages, unexplained mental handicap or malformed children, and parental consanguinity should be asked about specifically.

Investigations may involve chromosomal or DNA analysis or specific biochemical tests related to the disease being screened for.

Presenting the risks in context

Once the diagnosis and mode of inheritance have been established, carrier risk and recurrence risk for the consultands can be estimated, based on Mendelian rules and Bayes' theorem. In general, a risk greater than one in ten is considered to be high and a risk of less than one in 20 is considered to be low.

Discussing options, communication, and support

The counsellor must aim to be non-judgemental and non-directive towards the consultands when discussing their future options. At best, the counsellor can give the consultand reassurance that the recurrence risk is no greater than the population risk. If the recurrence risk is high, the counsellor must explore the feelings of the consultand towards the disease in terms of the emotional, physical, and financial implications. With these in mind the counsellor can provide information about the options open to them such as:

• No further pregnancies—advice about reliable forms

of contraception should be given.
• Prenatal diagnosis—selective termination of affected fetuses (see p. 132).
• Artificial insemination of donor sperm (AID)—if the male has an AD condition or both partners are carriers for an AR condition.
• Ignoring the risk and coping if an affected child is born

Follow-up sessions should be offered and the consultands should be kept on a register so they can be recalled if new prenatal or carrier tests are developed.

Ethical considerations in genetic counselling

Consanguinity and incest

Incest is the mating of first degree relatives. It has been outlawed in most human societies because of its risk of serious genetic disease (AR disorders). In the UK, double first cousins are the closest relatives allowed to marry (i.e. the two sets of parents are both full siblings) (Fig. 6.30). The risk of disease or serious congenital malformation in a child born to first cousins is 1 in 20. This rises to 1 in 11 in a highly inbred family. Therefore a detailed anomalies scan is indicated during the pregnancy as well as careful monitoring during and after the pregnancy.

Disputed paternity

Paternity testing uses modern DNA fingerprinting techniques. It is based on the detection of variable number tandem repeats (VNTRs) in genomic DNA. These are a series of allelic polymorphisms created by tandem arrangements of multiple copies of short DNA sequences. In DNA fingerprinting, the genomic DNA is cut with a frequent cutting restriction enzyme and a probe added that highlights the VNTR alleles. The fragment sizes are unique for each individual and the probability that two unrelated people have the same fragment pattern is less than 3×10^{-11} when one probe is used. Parents give half their VNTRs to their offspring so this test can be used to establish a child's parentage reliably.

Confidentiality and conflicts of interest

The laws of patient confidentiality must never be forgotten. This can sometimes be a problem if a family has a disease with a very clear pattern of inheritance and only some members of the family want to know their risks of being affected. Fig. 6.31 shows an example of a conflict of interest.

There are DNA analysis tests available that could be used to find out if the daughter is affected. These may not be very specific for her mutation so a negative result would not completely rule out her being affected. Linkage analysis using her father's

DNA would probably be more sensitive. On the other hand, if the DNA test shows she is positive, it would imply that her father is also positive and is likely to develop the disease before she does. If he does not want to know this, her attendance at counselling may create family tension.

- **Explain the probability theory as applied to genetics.**
- **Show how to calculate carrier and affected risks using mendelian inheritance.**
- **Outline the general aspects of genetic counselling.**
- **Describe some of the ethical considerations in genetic counselling.**

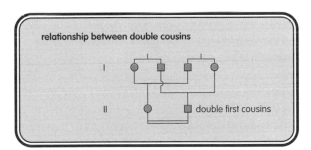

Fig. 6.30 Relationship between double first cousins.

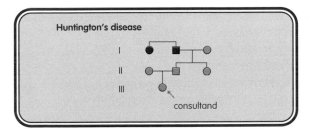

Fig. 6.31 Huntington's disease. The grandfather and his sister both died of Huntington's disease. The father is now in his late 30s and is still unaffected. The daughter (consultand) is now 19 years old and wants to know if she is affected.

POPULATION GENETICS AND SCREENING

Principles of population genetics
Allele frequencies in populations

Allele frequencies vary and are characteristic of different populations. Allele frequencies within a population tend to remain constant from one generation to the next, provided that:

- The population is large.
- There is random mating.
- The mutation rate remains constant.
- Alleles are not selected for.
- There is no migration into or out of the population.

Hardy–Weinberg principle

The Hardy–Weinberg law is a mathematical equation that forms the basis of population genetics.

In a gene pool, consider two alleles for a gene locus. Allele A has a frequency of p and allele a has a frequency of q such that

$$q = 1 - p$$

(A is the dominant allele; a is the recessive allele; Fig. 6.32.)

129

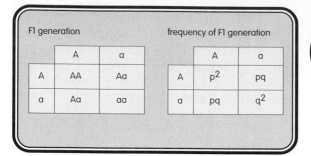

Fig. 6.32 The Hardy–Weinberg equation. Consider if two heterozygotes mate, Aa×Aa. The distribution of AA, Aa, and aa genotypes in the population correspond to p^2, $2pq$, and q^2, respectively. If A and a are the only alternative alleles for the same gene locus, then, $p^2 + 2pq + q^2 = 1$. (a, recessive allele; A, dominant allele; p, frequency of A; q, frequency of a.)

Learn this sentence!
Population screening aims to detect healthy people with a predisposition for a certain disease and intervene to slow down the course of the disease or prevent it altogether.

The Hardy-Weinberg equation is as follows (see Fig. 6.32):

$$p^2 + 2pq + q^2 = 1$$

This can be used to calculate allele frequency in a population if disease occurrence is known, provided that allele frequencies remain in equilibrium from one generation to the next.

For AR conditions, (incidence = q^2; gene frequency =q; heterozygote frequency = $2pq$ (e.g. cystic fibrosis):
- Incidence, $q^2 = 1/1600$.
- Gene frequency (a), q = 1/40; dominant allele A has gene frequency p = 39/40
- Heterozygote frequency, $2pq$ is $2 \times 39/40 \times 1/40$, which is approximately 1/20.

For AD conditions:
- Nearly all affected are heterozygotes, so q^2 is approximately 0.
- If the condition is rare, p^2 is approximately 1.
- Disease gene frequency (A) is approximately $2pq$, which is approximately 2q.

Genetic polymorphism in a population

Polymorphisms are different forms of the same allele in a population. The frequency of the rarer allele must be at least 0.01 for it to be considered to be a polymorphism rather than a recurrent mutation. The alleles of the ABO blood group system are examples of genetic polymorphisms.

Concepts of screening

A genetic disease is suitable for screening if it fulfils the following criteria:
- Clearly defined disorder.
- Appreciable frequency.
- Advantage to early diagnosis.
- Few false positives (specificity).
- Few false negatives (sensitivity).
- Benefits outweigh the costs.

Carrier detection and pre-symptomatic diagnosis
Linkage to polymorphic marker

Genetic linkage is the tendency for alleles close together on the same chromosome to be transmitted together through meiosis (i.e. they do not separate at crossing over in prophase of meiosis I, see Chapter 5). It allows disease genes for which markers have not yet been discovered to be followed through generations, using a detectable linked marker that lies near the disease gene. The marker is often a restriction fragment length polymorphism (RFLP) or 'polymerase chain reaction (PCR) minisatellite site' (i.e. a sequence containing a repeated di-, tri-, or tetranucleotide element of variable length, Fig. 6.33). Linkage allows the detection of familial diseases such as cystic fibrosis.

Biochemical tests

Biochemical tests form an important part of prenatal and pre-symptomatic diagnosis. Over 100 inborn errors of metabolism can be detected by fetal enzyme assays using cultured amniocytes or chorionic villus samples. Newborn babies can be screened for errors of metabolism by simple biochemical tests on a blood sample.

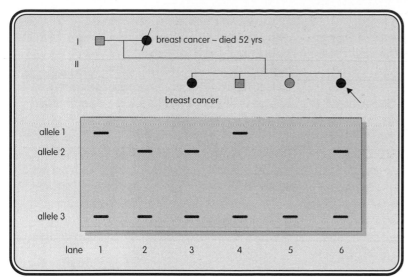

Fig. 6.33 Detection of inherited breast cancer using minisatellite linkage. Using a PCR minisatellite site known to be linked to the disease gene locus, three main alleles have been detected (each corresponding to a different repeat element). The affected mother has handed the disease gene and allele 2 to the affected daughter (lane 3) and her normal gene and allele 3 to each unaffected child (lanes 4 and 5). This could be a scenario where the mother and daughter have already both developed breast cancer and the test shows that the youngest daughter (lane 6) also has the disease gene so is at high risk of developing cancer. She should therefore have regular mammograms for early detection.

Tests used for prenatal diagnosis				
Test	**Gestation**	**Procedure**	**Abnormalities detected**	**Risk of procedure**
amniocentesis	16–18 weeks	liquor is removed via a long needle inserted transabdominally	fetal sexing, karyotyping, and enzyme assay	miscarriage rate estimated at 1% above the normal rate at 16 weeks
chorionic villus sampling	8–10 weeks	biopsy usually taken transabdominally or transvaginally	fetal sexing, fetal karyotyping, biochemical studies, DNA analysis (cell culture not necessary)	miscarriage rate estimated at 2–3% above the average at 10 weeks; rhesus isoimmunization if mother is rhesus negative
cordocentesis	18 weeks +	fetal blood sample obtained by inserting a fine needle into fetal umbilical cord	suspected fetal infection or mosaicism, unexplained hydrops, single gene disorders, fragile X	procedure-related loss approximately 1%; risk of rhesus isoimmunization
ultrasound	routine scan at 16–18 weeks in all pregnancies	visualization of fetus by transabdominal ultrasound probe	over 280 congenital malformations	non-invasive test with low associated risk
maternal serum screening: infectious screen (TORCH screen), triple test (serum AFP, HCG, and oestradiol)	16–18 weeks	sample of maternal blood collected	detection of infections that may cause congenital malformations (see Chapter 8); triple test estimates relative risk of NTDs and Down syndrome based on serum levels of HCG, AFP, and oestradiol	very low

Fig. 6.34 Some of the tests available in prenatal diagnosis.(AFP, α-fetoprotein; HCG, human chorionic gonadotrophin; NTDs, neural tube defects; TORCH, toxoplasmosis, other agents, rubella, cytomegalovirus, herpes simplex; NTD, neural tube defect. Associated risk refers to the risk that the test may damage the fetus.

Phenylketonuria (PKU) is routinely screened for in all newborn babies. Following its detection, the amino acid phenylalanine is excluded from the diet and this prevents the development of symptoms. A sample of blood is taken from a heel prick from all newborn babies. The blood is placed on a Guthrie card and used to detect PKU, congenital hypothyroidism, and galactosaemia.

Prenatal diagnosis

Fig. 6.34 describes some of the tests available in prenatal diagnosis and their relative risk to the pregnancy.

Population screening

Population screening is the screening of all members of a population regardless of their family history.

Carrier detection

This aims to isolate asymptomatic heterozygotes for AR traits. If two partners are heterozygotes for a mutation at the same locus, genetic counselling should be given before conception and prenatal tests offered as appropriate. Carrier detection tends to be confined to small ethnic populations in which there is an anomalously high incidence of a particular disease due to the founder effect, where one or more founder members of a small group carry a mutation and pass it on to their descendants.

Thalassaemia

Carrier detection of β thalassaemia is undertaken for Mediterranean populations and populations of South East Asia by finding a microcytosis—mean corpuscular volume (MCV) less than 75 fl with a low mean corpuscular haemoglobin (MCH) less than 25 pg and an increased haemoglobin A$_2$ concentration.

Sickle cell disease

Carrier detection is by the Sickledex test, which demonstrates sickling of red blood cells *in vitro* at very low oxygen concentrations. This test is targeted at US and African Blacks.

Tay–Sachs disease

Carriers are detected by measurement of serum β *N*-acetylhexosaminidase and the test is targeted at the Ashkenazi Jewish population (see p. 160).

Cystic fibrosis

Cystic fibrosis is the commonest serious AR condition to affect Caucasians. Carrier detection is limited to affected families and uses linkage studies or PCR, depending upon the character of the mutation. In some areas of the UK, cystic fibrosis is screened for at birth with PKU, hypothyroidism, and galactosaemia.

General population screening tests

These are usually quick and simple tests that can be used to assess a woman's relative risk of having an affected child. Maternal serum is used in many of these tests. At 16–18 weeks' gestation, women can be tested for maternal serum α-fetoprotein (MSAFP), human gonadotrophin (HCG), and oestradiol. These variables can be used to assess the relative risk of a number of fetal conditions.

Trisomy 21 and other chromosomal abnormalities

The detection of Down syndrome combines MSAFP and maternal age to form a combined risk (Fig. 6.35). MSAFP and HCG are also disturbed in other chromosomal abnormalities:

- MSAFP is low in trisomies 21, 18, and 13, and normal in X chromosomal abnormalities.
- HCG is high in trisomy 21, low in trisomy 18, and normal in trisomy 13 and X abnormalities.

Neural tube defects

Neural tube defects are associated with a high MSAFP because more of the fetal protein leaks into the amniotic fluid because of the malformation. As part of the routine 16–18-week check, pregnant women are referred for a detailed ultrasound scan if the MSAFP is on the 95th centile or above. Other conditions associated with a high MSAFP at 16–18 weeks are:

- Missed abortion.
- Oesophageal atresia.

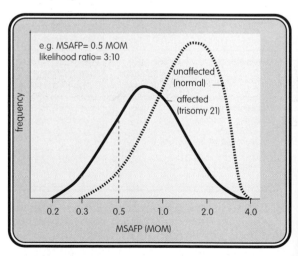

Fig. 6.35 Screening for trisomy 21. MSAFP levels are used to generate likelihood ratios, which are derived from overlapping distribution of affected and unaffected pregnancies. Likelihood ratio and maternal age are used together to generate a combined risk. If there is a high combined risk, refer for amniocentesis. If there is a low combined risk, provide reassurance. (MOM, multiples of the median.)

- Exomphalos.
- Sacrococcygeal teratoma.
- Bladder neck obstruction.
- Fetal–maternal haemorrhage.

'Cascade' screening

Within an extended family where an AR disorder or a late-onset AD disorder, has been diagnosed, those at highest risk are first offered definitive testing. The results are used to identify further family members at risk who are then offered the test. These results, in turn, redefine risk status for other members of the family—and so on.

- Describe the following principles of population genetics: allele frequencies, Hardy–Weinberg equation, genetic polymorphisms.
- What is meant by screening? Include ethical implications and types of screening.
- What is carrier detection and pre-symptomatic diagnosis?
- Give examples of prenatal diagnosis.
- What is population screening?

- Cleavage at specific sites using restriction endonucleases.
- Nucleic acid hybridization using Watson–Crick base pairing.
- DNA cloning.
- Sequencing often using automated sequencers.
- DNA engineering—manufacturing DNA by ligating fragments together, including the generation of transgenic animals.

Restriction endonucleases

These are enzymes that recognize specific sequences of DNA and cut it in a particular way, often creating overhanging 'sticky' ends, which can allow unrelated DNA fragments to be joined together (Fig. 6.36).

Ligases

Ligases can join together two pieces of DNA by forming a 3'–5' phosphodiester bond. They can be used to join together fragments generated by restriction enzymes.

DNA cloning

Cloning means producing identical copies of an object. DNA cloning plays a very important role in modern genetic techniques. The relevant DNA can be put into a self-replicating unit or vector that contains an origin of replication so can be replicated in a host cell. Fig. 6.37 summarizes the vectors that are commonly used and Fig. 6.38 shows the assembly and selection of a cosmid clone.

RECOMBINANT DNA TECHNOLOGY AS APPLIED TO MEDICINE

Overview

Recombinant DNA technology involves the manipulation of DNA using the following five techniques:

Recombinant DNA technology took off in the 1970s with the discovery of prokaryotic restriction endonucleases and ligases.

Examples of restriction endonucleases and their restriction sites	
Restriction endonucleases	**Restriction sites**
*Eco*RI	G↓AA*TTC, CTTAA↑G
Hpa II	C↓CGG, GGC↑C
Alu I	AG↓CT, TC↑GA
Tag I	T↓CGA*, AGC↑T

Fig. 6.36 Examples of some restriction endonucleases and their restriction sites. (A*, N⁶-methyladenine.)

Commonly used vectors			
Vector	**Origin**	**Features**	**Size of insert accommodated**
plasmid	circular double stranded DNA in the cytoplasm of bacteria; undergoes replication with the bacterial genome and is passed on through generations; can be regarded as bacterial parasites	origin of replication; antibiotic resistance genes; restriction enzyme site, which can break open plasmid and allow DNA to be inserted	less than 10 kb
phage	viruses that infect bacteria	phage particles can be assembled *in vitro*; DNA of interest is fragmented and ligated to phage *cos* sites; it is mixed with packaging extract, which contains all the proteins needed for phage assembly; phage heads are filled with DNA between two *cos* sites and a phage tail is attached; the assembled phage infects the host cell	16 kb
cosmid	a genetically engineered hybrid of a plasmid and a phage	contains plasmid origin of replication, selectable marker and phage *cos* site; assembly is in Fig. 6.38	45 kb
YAC	'yeast artificial chromosomes' are genetically engineered units that can be replicated in yeast cells	contain the three DNA sequences essential for yeast chromosome function: telomeres (*TEL*), origin of replication (*ARS*), centromere (*CEN*)	> 100 kb

Fig. 6.37 The most commonly used vectors in DNA cloning. *cos* sites are cohesive ends in phage DNA which facilitate the packaging of DNA into phage particles (see Fig. 6.38).

DNA libraries and DNA probes

A DNA library is a collection of cloned DNA fragments ligated into vectors and stored in host cells. The DNA inserted into the vectors can be derived from genomic DNA or from messenger RNA (mRNA) that has been converted into complementary DNA (cDNA) by the retroviral enzyme, reverse transcriptase. cDNA contains only expressed sequences (exons) as the introns are removed by splicing, whereas genomic DNA contains exons, introns, and intergenic DNA. Comprehensive genomic DNA and cDNA libraries have been made from a wide range of species.

cDNA libraries can be 'enriched' for rare transcripts by hybridizing cDNA from a highly specialized cell line with mRNA from a less specialized line. mRNA–cDNA hybrids form for the commonly occurring species and the unpaired, rare cDNAs left are extracted and inserted into vectors.

Chromosome-specific libraries can be created from chromosomes sorted by an automated machine such as a fluorescence-activated cell sorter (FACS), which uses fluorescent markers to sort the chromosomes.

Various commercial libraries are available, such as the National Institute of Health (NIH) and the French CEPH genomic libraries, which are used in molecular genetic laboratories throughout the world.

DNA probing is a technique that relies on the annealing properties of nucleic acids. Any two pieces of single stranded DNA (ssDNA) or RNA will bind together to form duplexes if they have complementary sequences of around 20 bases or more by Watson–Crick base pairing.

Probes are important in gene detection and are often labelled with radioactive isotopes such as ^{32}P or with fluorescent tags (Fig. 6.39).

Polymerase chain reaction

The polymerase chain reaction (PCR) uses a temperature-resistant DNA polymerase called *Taq* pol to amplify a segment of DNA between two primers. It is a rapid and sensitive way of making large amounts of target DNA—in 25 cycles of reaction, the target DNA can be amplified a million-fold (2^{25}). The primers are oligonucleotides with sequences that are known to lie either side of the target DNA. They must contain at least 20 bases (to allow accurate annealing) and can be synthesized artificially (Figs 6.40 and 6.41).

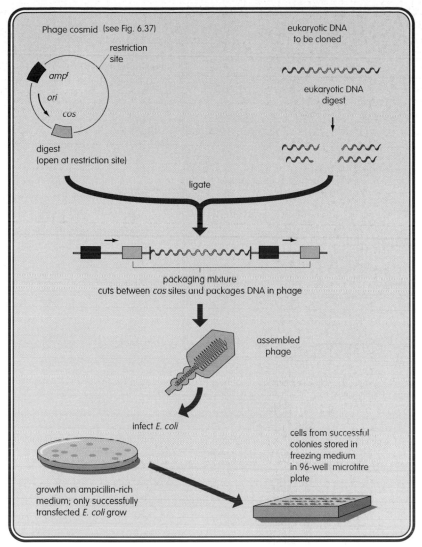

Phage cosmid (see Fig. 6.37)

restriction site

ampʳ

ori

cos

digest
(open at restriction site)

eukaryotic DNA
to be cloned

eukaryotic DNA
digest

ligate

packaging mixture
cuts between *cos* sites and packages DNA in phage

assembled
phage

infect *E. coli*

cells from successful
colonies stored in
freezing medium
in 96-well microtitre
plate

growth on ampicillin-rich
medium; only successfully
transfected *E. coli* grow

Fig. 6.38 Assembly and selection of a cosmid clone—*ampʳ* (ampicillin resistance gene) acts as a selectable marker for transfected cells. (*E. coli*, *Escherichia coli*; ori, origin of replication.) Cosmids are artificial plasmids derived from λ (lambda) phage DNA. *cos* stands for 'cohesive site' and this allows the cosmid to be packaged into a phage viral coat and cloned.

Methods of DNA analysis

In this section specific methods of DNA analysis are described with an emphasis on applications in medicine.

Restriction mapping

Restriction mapping is a way of using restriction enzymes to detect specific DNA sequences. DNA digested by a particular restriction enzyme will give a pattern of fragment sizes characteristic of the DNA sequence (Fig. 6.42).

Southern blotting

This is a way of transferring DNA from an electrophoresis gel onto a nitrocellulose membrane so that DNA is fixed. Probes can be applied to detect a specific DNA sequence (see Fig. 6.42).

DNA sequencing

Nucleotides of up to 500 base pairs can be sequenced by a chemical cleavage method (Maxam–Gilbert) or chain termination (Sanger) method. Both techniques are based on four reaction mixtures, each of which cleaves DNA at a specific base (i.e. adenine, cytosine, guanine, or thymine). The cleaved DNA is analysed by electrophoresis (Fig. 6.43).

Mutation screening techniques

These tests detect mutations without the exact nature of the mutation being known. The two tests outlined below are based on comparison of test and control DNA.

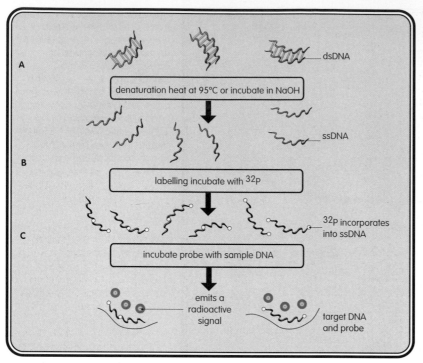

Fig. 6.39 Manufacture of a radioactive probe. (A) The target DNA is isolated and denatured. The source of the DNA may be synthetic, cDNA, or a restriction fragment. (B) ssDNA is labelled with [32]P. (C) The labelled probe will anneal to the complementary sequences in sample DNA.

Within Fig. 6.39:
- dsDNA
- denaturation heat at 95°C or incubate in NaOH
- ssDNA
- labelling incubate with [32]p
- [32]p incorporates into ssDNA
- incubate probe with sample DNA
- emits a radioactive signal
- target DNA and probe

A
B
C

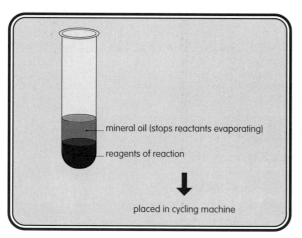

Within Fig. 6.40:
- mineral oil (stops reactants evaporating)
- reagents of reaction
- placed in cycling machine

Fig. 6.40 Reaction mixture contents for PCR. The reagents of reaction are template DNA; oligonucleotide primers (fragments that are complementary to 3' and 5' end of target DNA); nucleoside triphosphates—dATP (deoxyadenosine triphosphate), dCTP (deoxycytosine triphosphate), dGTP (deoxyguanosine triphosphate), dTTP (deoxythymidine triphosphate; DNA polymerase (*Taq* polymerase).

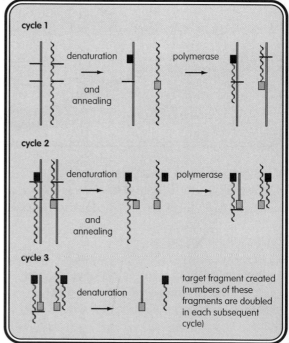

Within Fig. 6.41:
- cycle 1
- denaturation and annealing
- polymerase
- cycle 2
- denaturation and annealing
- polymerase
- cycle 3
- denaturation
- target fragment created (numbers of these fragments are doubled in each subsequent cycle)

Fig. 6.41 Mechanism of action of PCR. The typical cycling conditions are (1) 95°C for 5 min—denaturation of DNA to create ssDNA; (2) 60.5°C for 1 min—annealing of primer to target; (3) 72°C for 1 minute—polymerization (new strand of DNA formed); (4) and repeat for 35 cycles. Each primer anneals to a different strand.

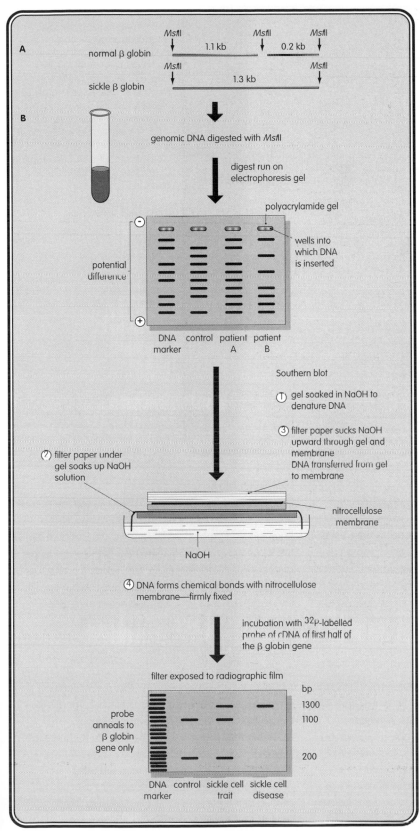

Fig. 6.42 Restriction mapping and Southern blotting using a clinical example of diagnosis of sickle cell disease, a point mutation in the gene for β haemoglobin which destroys a restriction site for *Msf*II. Genomic DNA is digested with *Msf*II and run on an electrophoresis gel. The gel separates the DNA fragments, making the small ones travel further. The DNA is stained with ethidium bromide and viewed under ultraviolet light. The DNA can be transferred onto nitrocellulose film by Southern blotting. (1) Gel soaked in NaOH to denature DNA. (2) The filter paper under gel soaks up NaOH solution. (3) The filter paper sucks NaOH upward through gel and membrane and so transfers DNA from gel to membrane. (4) DNA forms a chemical bond with nitrocellulose membrane and is firmly fixed. Radiolabelled probes on the Southern blot can be used to detect the β globin gene. The mutation is detected by a single large *Msf*II fragment. (Normal genes have two smaller *Msf*II fragments.)

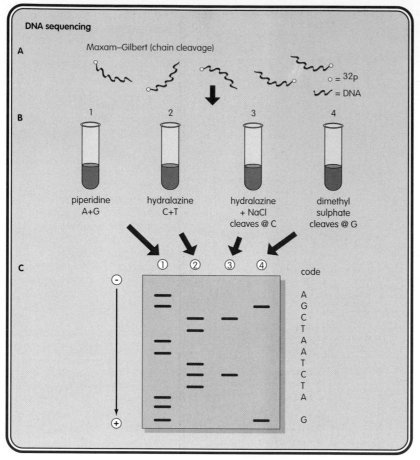

Fig. 6.43 Maxam–Gilbert method of DNA sequencing. (A) DNA fragments are end-labelled with ^{32}P. (B) Four reactions are set up. Each contains chemicals that cleave DNA at a specific base. (C) Fragments are separated by gel electrophoresis. The pattern of the fragments corresponds to the original base sequence because the pattern of cleavage was created by chemicals. (A, adenine; C, cytosine; G, guanine; T, thymine.)

Chemical cleavage mismatch (CCM)

Control and test DNA are generated by PCR. They are denatured and reannealed together. Osmium tetroxide is added, which will chemically alter incorrectly base paired duplex DNA. The altered bases are cleaved by piperidine. The treated DNA is separated by gel electrophoresis. If control and test DNA differ in sequence because of a mutation, greater than one fragment will be seen on the electrophoresis. The size of the fragments indicates the site of the mutation.

Protein truncation test (PTT)

This is the detection of nonsense mutations by identifying truncated protein products. Protein is generated from RNA collected from test and control cell lines. Its migration pattern on sodium dodecyl sulphate–polyacrylamide gel electrophoresis (SDS–PAGE; type of electrophoresis that separates proteins) will detect truncated products. This is a useful screening test for truncating mutations in large multi-exon genes such as dystrophin, which is associated with muscular dystrophies.

Northern blotting

This technique fixes RNA onto a nitrocellulose membrane in the same way that Southern blotting fixes DNA. Radiolabelled probes can be applied to a Northern blot in the same way as to a Southern blot. The intensity of the annealed probe reflects the level of transcription of the gene in the original cell. It can also detect tissue-specific expression of rare transcripts and detect truncated transcripts resulting from nonsense mutations.

Site-directed mutagenesis and transgenic animals

A DNA insert can be constructed that can alter the genome of a prokaryotic or eukaryotic cell. Specific sites in the genome can be targeted by homologous recombination (see meiosis). The insert may contain a 'reporter gene' attached to a sequence of DNA that corresponds to the gene being targeted. After homologous recombination a 'fusion protein' may be created that is easily identified in the cell so that the gene product's intracellular destination can be identified.

Fig. 6.44 Cystic fibrosis knock-out mouse.

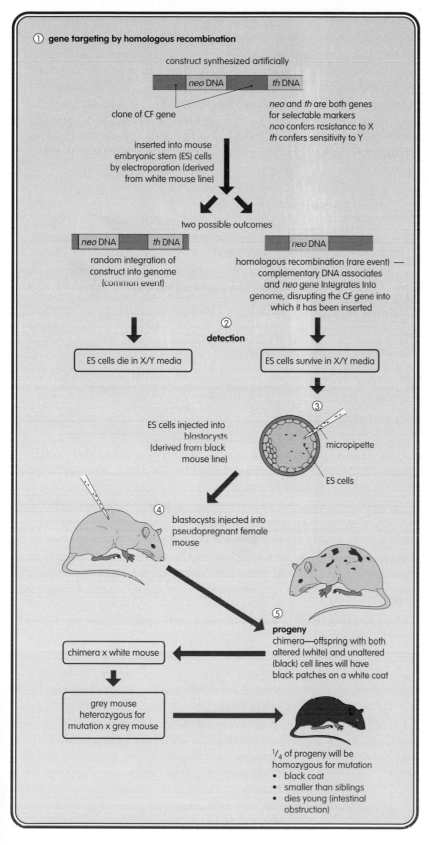

① **gene targeting by homologous recombination**

construct synthesized artificially

| neo DNA | th DNA |

clone of CF gene

neo and th are both genes for selectable markers
neo confers resistance to X
th confers sensitivity to Y

inserted into mouse embryonic stem (ES) cells by electroporation (derived from white mouse line)

two possible outcomes

| neo DNA | th DNA |

random integration of construct into genome (common event)

| neo DNA |

homologous recombination (rare event) — complementary DNA associates and neo gene integrates into genome, disrupting the CF gene into which it has been inserted

② **detection**

ES cells die in X/Y media

ES cells survive in X/Y media

③

micropipette

ES cells

ES cells injected into blastocysts (derived from black mouse line)

④ blastocysts injected into pseudopregnant female mouse

⑤ **progeny**
chimera—offspring with both altered (white) and unaltered (black) cell lines will have black patches on a white coat

chimera x white mouse

grey mouse heterozygous for mutation x grey mouse

$1/4$ of progeny will be homozygous for mutation
• black coat
• smaller than siblings
• dies young (intestinal obstruction)

139

A novel gene with its own control element can be inserted into a cell and may add into the genome randomly (i.e. not by homologous recombination; addition is a far more common event). The insert can code for 'anti-sense' RNA, which will bind to the sense RNA and prevent translation—this is one way of 'knocking out' a gene's function.

Gene targeting is a more sophisticated way of creating a gene 'knock-out.' This technique was used to create the 'knock-out mouse' model of cystic fibrosis (Fig. 6.44).

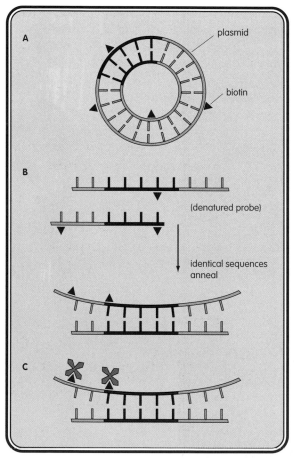

Fig. 6.45 Fluorescent probe manufacture. (A) The probe is labelled with biotin. It is generated in a plasmid and biotinylation is by nick translation where DNAase breaks through the plasmid and biotin inserts into defects (not shown in figure). (B) The plasmid is fragmented and denatured to produce an ssDNA biotinylated probe. (C) Avidin–fluorescein complex is added; the avidin binds to biotin with high affinity. The signal is amplified by addition of anti-avidin antibody, followed by more avidin (which binds to the anti-avidin antibody). The fluorescent signal from the fluorescein molecules is viewed directly under a fluorescent microscope (also not shown in figure).

Gene mapping and chromosome mapping

This is physical mapping of an organism's genome that aims to characterize its chromosomes in terms of the DNA sequence. This is done by establishing DNA 'landmarks' such as restriction sites and specific DNA sequences. The ultimate aim is to be able to describe every gene's position in terms of a comprehensive set of landmarks positioned at regular intervals along the chromosome. Genome projects exist for a number of species including yeast, sheep, and humans.

Somatic cell hybrids

This is a relatively crude way of characterizing DNA. One or more regions of human DNA are maintained and propagated in a rodent cell line. It is a way of mapping markers onto chromosome regions by finding which markers occur together on the same chromosome fragments.

In-situ hybridization

This technique is becoming increasingly important and is based on the annealing of identical sequences of DNA. Non-radioactive probes have been developed that can be viewed directly under a fluorescent microscope, making fluorescent in-situ hybridization (FISH) quick and safe (Fig. 6.45).

FISH applications
These include:

- Genome mapping. Biotinylated yeast artifical chromosomes (YACs) and cosmids are used as probes to identify their physical position in relation to the chromosome (the probe is added to metaphase chromosomes), and in relation to each other. Several labelled YACs or cosmids can simultaneously anneal to interphase nuclei to reveal their separation to within 50 kilobases. Alternatively, chromatin fibres can be denatured and extended on a microscope slide. Several non-overlapping labelled cosmids are added and their physical separation calculated, since 12 μm of fully extended chromatin is equivalent to 35 kilobases.
- Diagnosis of numerical chromosome abnormalities. Trisomies can be diagnosed by applying chromosome-specific fluorescent probes onto interphase nuclei and viewing the signal directly.
- Chromosome painting. An entire chromosome is isolated, fragmented, and the DNA labelled, then

added to a metaphase spread of the patient's chromosomes. Since the probe anneals to identical DNA, it can detect unusual chromosome rearrangements.

Chromosome walking and YAC contigs

Chromosome walking uses YACs and cosmids that have already been mapped as probes to find other clones that contain overlapping DNA sequences. The aim of chromosome walking is to create YAC or cosmid contigs, clones propagated in cloning vectors that create a contiguous series of slightly overlapping fragments corresponding to a large stretch of genomic DNA or RNA.

Contigs can be created using automated gridding procedures. Genomic/cDNA libraries stored in 96-well microtitre plates can be cultured in a high-density array on a nitrocellulose filter placed on nutrient agar. The high-density array is created using a 96-pin inoculating tool, which is operated by a programmable robotic arm. The arm can use the inoculating tool to transfer clones stored in the 96-well microtitre plates onto 16 different positions on the filter. Therefore over 20 000 clones can be cultured on the same agar plate (Fig. 6.46).

The clones are cultured for 3 hours and then the filter is removed from the plate and treated to:

- Lyse the cells.
- Remove all cellular proteins.
- Fix the DNA onto the filter.

Radiolabelled YACs and cosmids can then be applied to the filter to detect other clones with overlapping sequences (Fig. 6.47).

Gene therapy

Gene therapy is the transfer of new genetic material to the cells of an individual with the aim of therapeutic benefit to the individual. Requirements for gene therapy are as follows:

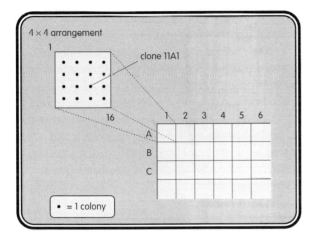

Fig. 6.46 4×4 arrangement of YAC/cosmid colonies on a high-density filter. Each dot corresponds to a separate colony. Each clone is named after its coordinates. Clone 11A1 is so named because of its position 11 in square A1.

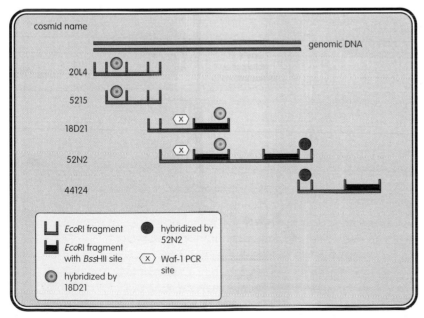

Fig. 6.47 Example of a cosmid contig (based on part of a contig created on chromosome 6 (6p21) *Eco*RI and *Bss*HII are restriction enzymes. 20L4, 5215, 18D21, etc., are names of cosmid clones. *Waf-1* is a gene which has an associated PCR site.

- Cloned disease gene from which functional copies have been made.
- A way of targeting the gene to affected tissues.
- It should not affect germ line cells so is not passed on to subsequent generations.
- Treatment should be given before irreversible pathology occurs (such as lung scarring in cystic fibrosis).

Genes are introduced into target cells or there is targeted destruction of gene product.

Over 100 clinical applications have been approved for gene therapy. Of these, less than 10% have been for genetic disease. Over 50% have been intended for the development of treatment for cancer.

Methods of DNA transfer can be viral or physical:

- Viral vectors are recombinant adenoviruses. The cloned gene is inserted in place of the viral E1 gene by homologous recombination (see Fig. 6.44). (The E1 gene codes for a protein vital for phage particle assembly.) Phage vectors are assembled in a cell line that expresses the E1 gene. The viral vectors are incapable of self-replication because they lack the E1 gene. The phage particles insert DNA into target cells in the same way as normal adenoviruses (see Fig. 5.48).
- Liposomes provide a physical method of DNA transfer. They are composed of a phospholipid bilayer arranged into a spherical micelle. DNA can be trapped inside the liposome or attached to its surface. Liposomes adhere to cell membranes and the DNA diffuses into the cell.

Cystic fibrosis (CF) is an autosomal recessive disease that causes gastrointestinal and lung problems (see Fig. 8.7). People with the condition usually die in their third decade from lung problems. The gene causing CF (*CFTR*) has been cloned and codes for a membrane chloride channel. CF has been selected as a promising target for gene therapy because introduction of the cloned gene into cultured *CFTR*-deficient cells corrects the chloride transfer defect. Also, lungs are a relatively accessible site for gene delivery. Adenovirus and liposome vectors have been used in clinical trials. Fig. 6.48 shows the advantages and disadvantages of *CFTR* delivery vectors.

CFTR delivery vectors: advantages and disadvantages		
Vector	**Advantages**	**Disadvantages**
recombinant adenovirus	targets the respiratory tract epithelium; infects non-replicating cells; in preliminary experiments 40% of respiratory epithelial cells took up the vector	expression in target cells transient; can create an inflammatory response in recipient; not known whether re-administration is safe (possibility of secondary immune response)
liposome	can be delivered directly to the lung (in an aerosol or by direct irrigation or intravenous infusion); re-administration is unlikely to cause an immune response	low uptake of liposomes: only 5% of epithelial cells transfected in preliminary experiments, which is not enough to have a therapeutic effect

Fig. 6.48 Advantages and disadvantages of *CFTR* delivery vectors

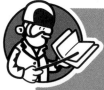

- What is DNA cloning? Describe with examples what is meant by a vector.
- What is a DNA library and how can probes be used to detect genes in DNA libraries?
- What is the polymerase chain reaction?
- Give a short account of restriction mapping and Southern blotting.
- Outline the principles involved in the creation of transgenic animals.
- Describe how genes can be mapped using cosmid and YAC contigs.
- What is meant by gene therapy? Outline the principles involved.

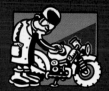

7. The Genetic Consultation

GENETIC CONSULTATION AND HISTORY TAKING

Things to remember when taking a history

The following points are very important when taking a history:

- Always introduce yourself.
- When dealing with children, provide a toy to distract them while discussing the case with the parents.
- Look around the bedside (where appropriate) for clues: inhaler, oxygen, walking stick or frame.
- Watch the patient for clues while taking the history, for example agitation or distress; can you see any tremors, twitches, or behavioural abnormalities. How does the patient interact with his or her family?

Structure of the genetic consultation
Some important points

An accurate diagnosis is essential if relevant genetic advice is to be given. It is important that information is given in a way that the consultands (people receiving the advice) can understand. It is useful to ask them what they understand about genetics before attempting to explain the nature of the disease. For example, do they understand what a chromosome or a gene is? This may also be useful in finding out whether they attach any stigma to the disease, such as self-blame or anger.

Counselling should be non-judgemental and non-directive. The counsellor should aim to make the consultands aware of the risk of having an affected child, the possible means of prevention including prenatal diagnosis and carrier detetion, and treatment of the disease. The counsellor must never sway the opinions of the consultands.

Outline of the interview
Presenting complaint

Are the symptoms felt by the patient or noticed by the parents?

In a genetic history, the family history is of paramount importance and may be discussed first.

History of the presenting complaint

Allow the patient (or more often the parents) to talk about what they perceive to be the problem; find out what they expect from the consultation and their concerns. Ask about:

- The nature of the complaint.
- Extent of any deficit.
- The onset and time course of the complaint.
- The pattern: constant or intermittent, frequency, duration.
- Precipitating and relieving factors.
- Other relevant symptoms.
- Any previous treatment or investigations for this complaint.

Family history

Particular attention should be given to relatives with relevant disorders. A family tree should be constructed to show how the condition has been passed on through the family. A standardized set of symbols is used, as described in Fig. 6.1. The male line is conventionally placed on the left and members of the same generation are placed on the same horizontal level. An arrow is used to indicate the proband (affected individual whose diagnosis caused the consultands to seek advice).

Enquire specifically about:

- Infant deaths, stillbirths, and abortions as this may alter recurrence risks (e.g. spina bifida is associated with an increased risk of neural tube defect in subsequent children).
- Consanguinity.
- Illegitimacy (discreetly!), as this may explain unexpected disease incidences.

Take information from both sides of the family—this may reveal useful information and avoids guilt or blame directed at one person. Record:

- Dates of birth rather than ages.
- Women's maiden names—this may help reveal cases of maternal transmission.
- Addresses of relevant family members.

An accurate family tree should reveal the mode of inheritance of the genetic disease and its penetrance and possibly where it originated from in the first place. In this way, realistic risk calculations can be made for the family with regard to future pregnancies (see Chapter 6).

Social history

The social history may have relevance to the consultand's reproductive choices. Relevant details include marital status, children, religious beliefs, occupational history, accommodation, diet, exercise, and risk behaviours such as smoking and alcohol.

Past medical history

Previous medical conditions should be enquired about where appropriate. Past medical history should also include obstetric history (e.g. maternal health, teratogen exposure, viral infections).

Drug history

Details of all prescription and over-the-counter drugs, any known allergies, and exposure to toxins such as alcohol, tobacco, or industrial toxins should be obtained.

Review of the systems

There should be an emphasis on finding any conditions that may have a genetic component or be suggestive of a syndrome or an association (see Chapter 8) (Fig. 7.1).

Summary

Give a full summary when presenting the case.

Systems review	
System	**Things to ask about**
cardiovascular	congenital heart disease, hypertension, hyperlipidaemia, vessel disease, heart attacks, strokes
respiratory	recurrent lung infections, asthma, bronchitis
gastrointestinal	atresia (at any level), fistulas (e.g. tracheo-oesophageal), recurrent diarrhoea, chronic constipation
genitourinary	ambiguous genitalia, abnormal renal function
musculoskeletal	muscle wasting or weakness
neurological	developmental milestones, hearing, vision, coordination, fits

Fig. 7.1 Systems review in genetic history taking.

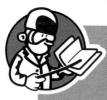

- **What should you remember when taking a history?**
- **List the some of the important points in the structure of the genetic consultation.**
- **Give an outline of the interview.**

COMMON PRESENTATIONS OF GENETIC DISEASE

Most syndromes and disorders mentioned in this section are further explained in Chapter 8.

Development
There are eight areas of childhood development:
- Hearing.
- Vision.
- Gross motor skills.
- Fine motor skills.
- Language comprehension.
- Expressive language.
- Behaviour and emotional development.
- Social skills.

These areas are interconnected and affect each other (e.g. difficulty in vision affecting fine motor skills).
In assessment, observation is divided into:
- Development rate (check whether within normal range).
- Pattern of development (qualitative rather than quantitative milestones observed).
- Final level of attainment (e.g. adult IQ level).

Deviations in development
Deviations can be the result of abnormalities in any of the areas listed above.

Hearing loss
Hearing loss can be conductive or sensorineural. Conductive deafness in childhood is rarely directly genetic. Sensorineural deafness is uncommon and is not always genetic (see p. 147).

Vision
In 50% of cases, visual impairment has genetic causes (see p. 146).

Gross motor skills
Conditions that affect muscle tone or nerve supply will impair gross motor skills (see p. 148). The quality of the movement can be affected, the child may fall over, or there may be a regression of motor skills.

Fine motor skills
These are also affected by neuromuscular problems, but it should be remembered that vision has a large impact on this developmental category.

Behaviour development and social skills
There are specific genetic syndromes that have characteristic behaviour patterns. For example:
- Gregarious personality—Williams syndrome.
- Inappropriate laughter with absent speech—Angelman's syndrome.
- Motor and vocal tics—Gilles de la Tourette syndrome.

Many genetic conditions have an effect on behavioural development due to the complicated impact of factors including hospitalization, decreased IQ, illness behaviour, stigmatization, and coping with a chronic illness.
Language is affected by all the above eight areas of development and is assessed in the two areas of:
- Speech (vocal sounds made).
- Language (comprehension and expression).

An example of the effect that a genetic disease can have on language development is Down syndrome where:
- Low IQ affects language comprehension.
- Conductive deafness due to secretory otitis media affects speech and language.
- Macroglossia affects sound production.

Failure to thrive
Failure to thrive is defined as suboptimal growth and weight gain in infants and toddlers. It is usually detected when values plotted on a centile chart begin to cross centile lines. Many childhood conditions are first diagnosed when the child presents with failure to thrive. Causes can be divided into organic and non-organic (environment deprivation).
Genetic causes of organic failure to thrive are:
- Decreased food intake. This can be primary (e.g. inability to feed due to cleft palate) or secondary to chronic illness (e.g. cystic fibrosis).
- Decreased food absorption (e.g. due to cystic fibrosis causing pancreatic insufficiency).

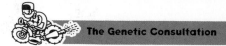

- Increased energy requirements (e.g. due to cystic fibrosis).
- Metabolic disorders (e.g. mucopolysaccharidoses).
- Miscellaneous causes including chromosomal disorders and syndromes.

Oral and facial deformities

Abnormal facies are common in genetic conditions so it is important to make accurate measurements of the facial landmarks if an abnormality is suspected (e.g. interpupillary distance). Craniofacial syndromes can be described using the terms:

- Hypertelorism—increased interpupillary distance.
- Hypotelorism—decreased interpupillary distance.
- Low-set ears—upper border of ear attachment is below level of inner corner of the eye (inner canthus).
- Mongoloid slant—inner canthi are below outer canthi.
- Antimongoloid slant—outer canthi below inner canthi.
- Epicanthic folds—skin folds over inner canthi.
- Brachycephaly—short anteroposterior skull length.

Examples of craniofacial malformations include:

- Cleft lip and palate—seen in many syndromes of mendelian inheritance (e.g. chondrodysplasia punctata), chromosomal disorders (e.g. trisomy 13), and non-mendelian syndromes (e.g. Pierre Robin syndrome—cleft palate with mandibular hypoplasia).
- Craniosynostosis—premature fusion of sutures can be due to genetic syndromes (e.g. Crouzon syndrome).
- Treacher Collins syndrome—hypoplasia of the mandible, with antimongoloid slant of eyes, deformed ears in 80%, and deafness in 40%.
- Sturge–Weber syndrome—haemangiomatous facial lesion (port wine stain) in ophthalmic division of trigeminal nerve distribution. Haemangiomatous extension into the brain may cause epilepsy, learning difficulties, and paralysis. It is almost always sporadic.

Although not a malformation, it should be noted that abnormal head circumference is associated with some genetic conditions. For example:

- Microcephaly reflects decreased brain growth as seen in cases of severe learning difficulties.
- Macrocephaly is seen in CNS storage disorders (e.g. mucopolysaccharidoses).

Eye disorders
Choroidoretinal degenerations

These include:

- Retinitis pigmentosa—autosomal recessive in 80%, autosomal dominant in 15%, and X-linked in 5% (but 50% of males). It is normally isolated, but can be part of a syndrome.
- Night blindness—usually autosomal dominant and isolated.

Nystagmus

Causes of nystagmus may be primary ocular disease or nystagmus may be secondary to neurological or vestibular disorders. Ocular albinism is an example and is X-linked recessive.

Other eye disorders

These include:

- Disorders of colour vision—all are X-linked recessive and occur in 8% of males. Because of the high expressivity, children of either sex can be affected (carrier female and affected male).
- Leber's optic atrophy—discussed under mitochondrial inheritance (see p. 115).
- Corneal dystrophies—require specialist opthalmological referral (e.g. clouding seen in mucopolysaccharidosis).
- Retinal detachment—commonly associated with high myopia. Genetic syndromes associated include Stickler syndrome.
- Retinoblastoma—discussed in Chapter 8 (see p. 168).
- Cataracts—congenital cataracts can be associated with syndromes (e.g. Down syndrome) and genetic metabolic disorders (e.g. mucopolysaccharidosis). Some genetic disorders can cause cataracts in later life (e.g. myotonic dystrophy, which is mendelian, and diabetes mellitus, which is polygenic).
- Kayser–Fleischer rings—due to copper accumulation in the cornea and seen in Wilson disease.
- Glaucoma—congenital glaucoma can be primary following autosomal recessive inheritance or associated with other syndromes (e.g. retinoblastoma, Sturge–Weber syndrome).
- Refractive errors—can be associated with syndromes (e.g. myopia and Marfan syndrome).
- Cyclops—all are lethal and sporadic (see p. 171).

- Microphthalmos and anophthalmos—both these abnomalities can be features of many chromosomal disorders (e.g. trisomy 13).
- Aniridia—may be associated with Wilms' tumour.
- Ptosis—may be isolated as an autosomal dominant disorder or may have a neuromuscular cause (e.g. myotonic dystrophy).

Ear disorders
Severe congenital sensorineural deafness
First exclude external factors such as rubella and cytomegalovirus infection. About 40–50% of genetic causes are due to autosomal recessive inheritance and 10% are due to autosomal dominant inheritance; X-linked inheritance is rare.

Partial nerve deafness
Some forms are present at birth while others are progressive. More than 10% have autosomal dominant inheritance, for example otosclerosis, which is a mixed conductive and neural deafness that has a progressive course and incomplete penetrance.

Syndromes associated with deafness
Waardenburg syndrome is associated with deafness and is autosomal dominant. The characteristics are a white forelock and decreased IQ. Alport's syndrome is also associated with deafness (see Chapter 8, Fig. 8.4).

External ear malformations
These can be related to syndromes (e.g. fragile X is associated with very large ears).

Skin disorders
These include:
- Ichthyoses—can be associated with syndromes (e.g. chondrodysplasia punctata—Conradi's syndrome).
- Epidermolysis bullosa—a heterogeneous group of disorders that can be autosomal dominant or recessive.
- Naevi—can be isolated autosomal dominant or associated with syndromes (e.g. Turner's syndrome). They must be distinguished from the lesions of tuberous sclerosis and neurofibromatosis, and pigmented lesions over spina bifida.
- Cavernous haemangiomas—usually sporadic (e.g. Sturge–Weber syndrome).
- Albinism—autosomal recessive. There are two main types attributable to mutations in different genes, which vary in their severity.
- Vitiligo—usually autosomal dominant.
- Acanthosis nigricans—primary acanthosis nigricans is autosomal dominant, but acanthosis nigricans can also be secondary to other disorders and may be acquired as a result of visceral malignancy.

Skin tumours
There are a number of very rare mendelian inherited skin tumours. Skin tumours may also result from genetic DNA repair disorders, for example, xeroderma pigmentosum (see Chapter 8, p. 168). Kaposi's sarcoma has an inherited form. Most cases of malignant melanoma are non-genetic, but an autosomal dominant predisposition has been described. Basal cell naevus syndrome (Gorlin's) syndrome predisposes to basal cell carcinoma (see p. 168).

Bone and connective tissue disorders
The following syndromes are discussed in Chapter 8:
- Achondroplasia.
- Marfan syndrome.
- Ehlers–Danlos syndrome.
- Mucopolysaccharidoses.
- Congenital dislocation of the hip.
- Talipes.

Other bone and connective tissue disorders are:
- Chondrodysplasia punctata—there is a characteristic facies with a saddle nose (nasal hypoplasia), frontal bossing, and a short stature. This syndrome is also characterized by cataracts, mental retardation, and ichthyoses.
- Lethal dysplasias—for example, thanatophoric dwarfism.
- Osteopetrosis—characterized by hard, dense, and brittle bones, described as 'marble bone' decease. Decreased marrow may result in anaemia and thrombocytopenia, and compression of cranial nerves may result in optic atrophy and deafness. The mild form is autosomal recessive; the severe form is autosomal dominant.
- Polydactyly (extra digits)—this can be isolated as an autosomal dominant condition or form part of a syndrome (e.g. trisomy 13; Ellis–van Creveld syndrome).

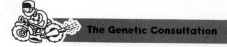

- Brachydactyly (short fingers)—generally this is autosomal dominant and associated with syndromes such as Turner's syndrome.
- Rockerbottom feet—a fat pad is increased on the sole. It is associated with trisomy 18.
- Limb reductions—these are associated with vertebral, anal, tracheo-oesophageal and renal (VATER) anomalies (see p. 176) and other syndromes.
- Osteogenesis imperfecta—brittle bone disease caused by a collagen defect: type 1 causes blue sclerae and deafness; type 2 is lethal; type 3 is characterized by fractures at birth with increasing deformity; type 4 is characterized by fragile bones and blue sclerae.

Neuromuscular disorders
Muscular dystrophies
There are many types of muscular dystrophies, the most important being X-linked Duchenne and Becker muscular dystrophies (see Fig. 8.8), and autosomal myotonic dystrophies (see p. 157). Muscular dystrophies present with muscular weakness and often progressive loss of motor milestones.

Spinal muscular atrophies
These are disorders of the anterior horn cell and present with weakness, wasting, and loss of reflexes. Most are autosomal recessive.

Hereditary motor sensory neuropathies
These present with progressive distal muscle wasting. They are usually of autosomal dominant inheritance (e.g. type I Charcot–Marie–Tooth disease, see Chapter 8).

Other neuromuscular disorders
These include:
- Myotonic disorders—present with delayed muscle relaxation (e.g. myotonic dystrophy, see pp. 157–8).
- Metabolic myopathies—present with floppiness, weakness, or cramps (e.g. glycogen storage disorders and mitochondrial cytopathies).

Central nervous system and psychiatric disorders
The following disorders are discussed in Chapter 8:
- Neural tube defects.
- Huntington's disease.

Other central nervous system disorders include:
- Rett syndrome—presents with deterioration in cognition, autistic behaviour, and stereotyped hand movement.
- Gilles de la Tourette syndrome—presents with tics.
- Ataxia—many syndromes present with ataxia, some of which are inherited, the commonest being Friedreich's ataxia (see Fig. 8.7), and ataxia telangiectasia (see p. 165).

Dementia
Dementia presents with a global impairment of higher cognitive function. Presenile dementia occurs before 65 years of age. It is most commonly caused by Alzheimer's disease which has an autosomal dominant inheritance and is also a feature of Down syndrome. Creutzfeldt–Jakob disease is a prior disease which can cause dementia.

Neurocutaneous syndromes
These are neurofibromatosis, tuberous sclerosis, and von Hippel–Lindau disease (see pp. 167–8).

Mental retardation
This is seen in a wide variety of genetic diseases and disorders frequently associated with mental retardation are:
- Autosomal dominant (e.g. Huntington's disease, myotonic dystrophy, neurofibromatosis, tuberous sclerosis).
- Autosomal recessive (e.g. ataxia telangiectasia, mucopolysaccharidoses, phenylketonuria).
- X-linked (e.g. fragile X syndrome).
- Chromosomal (e.g. Down syndrome, Klinefelter's syndrome, Turner's syndrome, Prader–Willi syndrome).
- Metabolic (e.g. Wilson's disease).

Schizophrenia
This has a genetic component (see p. 122).

Affective psychoses
These have multifactorial inheritance.

Behavioural disorders
Most behaviours are a combination of genetic and environmental factors, but some syndromes are associated with consistent behaviours (e.g. XYY syndrome and antisocial outbursts).

Disorders of thoracic development

These include:

- Pectus excavatum—seen in Noonan's syndrome.
- Wide nipples and shield-like chest—seen in Turner's syndrome.
- Gynaecomastia—seen in Klinefelter's syndrome.
- Kyphoscoliosis (anterior chest wall deformity)—seen in Marfan syndrome.
- Chest infection—seen in cystic fibrosis and α-1-antitrypsin deficiency.

Congenital heart disease

Examples include:

- Pulmonary stenosis and atrial septal defects in Noonan's syndrome.
- Aortic stenosis and pulmonary stenosis in Williams syndrome.
- Ventricular septal defect and patent ductus arteriosus in Edwards' syndrome or Patau's syndrome.
- Coarctation of the aorta in Turner's syndrome.
- Truncus arteriosus and pulmonary atresia in DiGeorge syndrome.
- Aortic incompetence and dissecting aortic aneurysm in Marfan syndrome.
- A cardiovascular abnormality (e.g. atrioventricular septal defects, patent ductus arteriosus, tetralogy of Fallot) in 40% of cases of Down syndrome.
- Ellis-van Creveld syndrome (polydactyly and CHD).

Other heart disorders

These include:

- Cardiomyopathies—may be seen in muscular dystrophies and Friedreich's ataxia.
- Coronary artery disease—familial hypercholesterolaemia accounts for 10% of early coronary artery disease.
- Hypertension—this is multifactorial.
- Dextrocardia and bronchiectasis—seen in Kartagener's syndrome, which is characterized by defective ciliary function and is autosomal recessive with 50% penetrance.

Gastrointestinal disorders

These include:

- Infantile pyloric stenosis—shows polygenic inheritance (see page. 174).
- Exomphalos and gastroschisis—exomphalos can be associated with Beckwith's syndrome, in which there is also macroglossia and hypoglycaemia.

Exomphalos is associated with major congenital abnormalities, while gastroschisis is not.

- Umbilical hernia—seen in Wilms' tumour.
- Bowel atresia—meconium ileus is seen in cystic fibrosis (not true atresia) and duodenal atresia is seen with increased frequency in Down syndrome.
- Peptic ulcer—has a multifactorial inheritance.
- Coeliac disease—associated with HLA-DR3 and HLA-B8.
- Intestinal polyposis—see Chapter 8.
- Imperforate anus—associated with VATER syndrome.
- Pancreatitis—this can be hereditary and is also seen in cystic fibrosis, both causing malabsorption and recurrent abdominal pain.

Liver disease

Metabolic liver disease presenting with cirrhosis, acute hepatitis, or portal hypertension is seen in Wilson disease, where there is aberrant copper deposition in the liver, brain, and cornea; it is inherited as an autosomal recessive disorder.

Other liver disorders include:

- Haemochromatosis—see Fig. 8.7.
- α-1-antitrypsin deficiency—an important cause of neonatal hepatitis and cirrhosis, with some adults developing emphysema. It is autosomal recessive.
- Hyperbilirubinaemias—present with jaundice and tend to result from enzyme deficiencies An example of this is Gilbert syndrome, which is often completely benign.
- Biliary atresia—presents in the infant with persistent jaundice and pale stools. Occasionally associated with chromosomal trisomies.
- Polycystic disease of the liver—isolated cases are autosomal recessive, but adult polycystic kidney disease (autosomal dominant) can be associated with a few hepatic cysts.

Genitourinary tract disorders

These include:

- Polycystic kidney disease—this commonly presents with deteriorating renal function, or the infantile form may be detected on routine antenatal ultrasound scan. There is an adult form (autosomal dominant) and a more severe infantile form (autosomal recessive). It can also be associated with trisomy 13, trisomy 18, tuberous sclerosis, and Meckel syndrome.
- Alport's syndrome—presents with microscopic

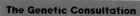

haematuria and sensorineural deafness (see Fig. 8.9).

- Fabry's disease—this X-linked disorder presents with angiokeratomas of the skin, numerous cardiac signs, and haematuria (see Fig. 8.8).
- Urinary malformation—this can be detected on antenatal ultrasound and causes obstruction or recurrent urinary tract infections.
- Renal stones—present with renal colic (excruciating intermittent back pain). Haematuria may be present. Most are not usually due to genetic causes, but they can be due to rare inherited metabolic disorders (e.g. cystinuria) and can occur more frequently in syndromes such as Lesch–Nyhan syndrome.
- Renal tumours—these present with haematuria, obstruction, or general ill health (cachexia and loss of appetite). Two important genetic renal tumours are Wilms' tumour and renal carcinoma associated with von Hippel–Lindau syndrome.
- Hypogonadism—this presents with infertility in either sex or reduced testicular volume in males. It may be isolated or part of a syndrome (Fig. 7.2).
- Macro-orchidism—greater than normal testicular volume and characteristic of fragile X syndrome (see p. 156).
- Virilized external genitalia (girls) or precocious puberty (boys)—these are the presentations of congenital adrenal hyperplasia, which occasionally presents as an emergency with a salt-losing crisis (see Fig. 8.7).

Recurrent abortions

These may result from parental or fetal factors. There may be an autosomal recessive lethal disorder (increased risk with consanguinity), an X-linked lethal disorder in the male, or a cytogenetic abnormality in the germ line (e.g. translocation). Fetal causes include a major abnormality such as neural tube defects or chromosomal disorders.

Inborn errors of metabolism

These may present with metabolic acidosis, unusual body odours, hypoglycaemia, respiratory distress, jaundice, urea and electrolyte imbalance, diarrhoea, failure to thrive, lethargy, fits, and coma. Most are mendelian (autosomal recessive). Examples include porphyrias, mucopolysaccharidoses, phenylketonuria, Tay–Sachs disease, Gaucher disease, and aminoacidurias.

Blood disorders

These include:

- Sickle cell disease—may present with failure to thrive, neonatal jaundice, or crises (see Fig. 8.7). It can be detected by prenatal diagnosis or screening.
- Thalassaemia—may present with anaemia, neonatal jaundice, or stillbirth (see Fig. 8.7). It may be detected by prenatal diagnosis or screening.
- Glucose-6-phosphate deficiency—may present with neonatal jaundice or haemolysis precipitated by drugs or fava beans (see Fig. 8.8).
- Fanconi's syndrome—may present with a pancytopenia.
- Immunodeficiencies—may present with recurrent infections, for example X-linked Bruton's agammaglobulinaemia or, less commonly, severe combined immunodeficiency (SCID) (see Fig. 8.9) and ataxia telangiectasia (see p. 165).
- Coagulation disorders—may present with bleeding e.g. haemophilia A and B (Fig. 8.8) and von Willebrand disease (Fig. 8.6).

Hypogonadism as part of a syndrome	
Male	**Female**
Klinefelter syndrome (XXY)—usually sporadic	Turner's syndrome (XO)—usually sporadic
Kallmann syndrome (hypogonadotrophic hypogonadism with anosmia)—X-linked recessive	XX gonadal dysgenesis—autosomal recessive (sex limited)
Reifenstein syndrome (hypogonadism with hypospadias)—X-linked recessive	XY gonadal dysgenesis—X-linked recessive
Prader–Willi (hypogonadism with obesity, hypotonia, small hands and feet)—usually sporadic (risk to siblings 1–2%)	testicular feminization (complete and incomplete)—X-linked recessive

Fig. 7.2 Hypogonadism as part of a syndrome.

○ **What are the eight areas of childhood development?**
○ **List (at least five) of the genetic disorders of the eye, the ear, bone and connective tissue, central nervous system (including psychiatric), gastrointestinal tract, genitourinary tract, and blood.**

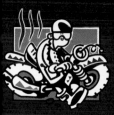

8. Examples of Genetic Disease

Introduction

Chromosomal disorders may arise from an error in:

- Female gametogenesis.
- Male gametogenesis.
- Fertilization.
- Cleavage of the zygote.

Of all conceptions, 7.5% involve a chromosomal disorder and 0.6% survive to birth; most chromosomal disorders result in a very early (less than 12 weeks) spontaneous abortion.

Chromosomal disorders are either numerical or structural:

- Numerical disorders are usually due to non-disjunction or anaphase lag. Non-disjunction means that the chromosomes or sister chromatids fail to separate. This usually occurs at anaphase II. Anaphase lag means that there is a delayed movement of a chromosome to the pole at anaphase and the chromosome is therefore excluded from the daughter cell nucleus.
- Structural disorders may be due to translocation, deletion, a ring chromosome, duplication, inversion, an isochromosome, or centric fragments.

Examples of numerical chromosomal disorders

Some examples of numerical chromosomal disorders are:

- Down syndrome (Fig. 8.1).
- Trisomy 18 and trisomy 13 (Fig. 8.2).

Triploidy means there are three whole sets of chromosomes. Trisomy means there are three copies of a particular chromosome. Other important definitions include:

- **Heteroploidy: any chromosome number other than normal.**
- **Aneuploidy: fewer or more chromosomes than an exact multiple of the haploid set.**
- **Polyploidy: three or more entire sets of chromosomes.**

Features, diagnosis, and prognosis of Down syndrome			
Disorder	**Features**	**Diagnosis**	**Prognosis**
trisomy 21 (Down syndrome); 1 in 650 liveborns; extra chromosome 21; age of mother affects probability of having Down syndrome baby —1 in 1000 probability for 25–30-year-old mothers, but 1 in 40 probability for 45-year-old mothers	facial: slanty eyes (mongoloid—pointing out and up), epicanthic folds, Brushfield spots on iris, flat round face, flat occiput, brachycephalic skull, low-set ears, protruding tongue; other—dermatoglyphics (abnormal palmar and plantar creases, including single palmar [simian] crease); congenital heart disease in 46% (lack endocardial cushion); duodenal atresia (bile-stained vomit); mental retardation IQ < 50 (but highly variable); later—lymphoblastic leukaemia (1%), Alzheimer's disease by 30–40 years of age, small stature, respiratory infections, secretory otitis media, cataracts and squints (2%), hypothyroid (3%), epilepsy (10%), diabetic risk increased, early onset atheromatous degeneration of the CVS	diagnosis is obvious by facial appearance alone in 90%; chromosome analysis is definitive; prenatal diagnosis is available—screening of women > 35 years only includes 10% of the pregnant population; improved strategy combines age, maternal serum AFP (MSAFP), unconjugated oestradiol and HCG to give a composite risk —this screening system has a 60% detection rate	cardiac defects can lead to death in infancy; presenile dementia > 40 years; usually life expectancy is less than 50 years

Fig. 8.1 Features, diagnosis, and prognosis of Down syndrome.

Sex chromosome abnormalities

Examples of sex chromosome abnormalities are:
- Klinefelter's syndrome (Fig. 8.3).
- Turner's syndrome (Fig. 8.3).

XXX

This is a female with an extra X chromosome and has an incidence of 1 in 1500 females; 25% are infertile and some have mild mental retardation, but there are no distinguishing features.

XYY

This male has an extra Y chromosome, the incidence being 1 in 1000 males. XYY males are often tall, but have

Features of trisomy 18 and trisomy 13			
Disorder	**Features**	**Diagnosis**	**Prognosis**
trisomy 18 (Edwards' syndrome); incidence 1 in 8000 live births; aetiology—extra chromosome 18	elongated skull, small jaw, low-set malformed ears with large lobes, congenital heart disease, malformed kidneys, clenched hands, rockerbottom feet, developmental delay	suspected clinically, confirmed by chromosome analysis	90% die within the first years, most in first few weeks
trisomy 13 (Patau syndrome); incidence 1 in 14 000 live births; aetiology—extra chromosome 13	severe bilateral cleft lip (+/− cleft palate), narrow temples, deformed ears and deafness, structural brain defect, congenital heart disease, malformed kidneys, polydactyly (extra digits), malformed small widely set eyes (eyes may be absent)	clinical suspicion confirmed by chromosomal analysis	most die within hours to days

Fig. 8.2 Features of trisomy 18 and trisomy 13.

Features of some sex chromosome abnormalities				
Disorder	**Aetiology**	**Features**	**Diagnosis**	**Prognosis**
Klinefelter syndrome; incidence 1 in 500 liveborn males	male XXY (47 chromosomes); extra maternal or paternal chromosome; incidence is increased in infertile male populations	female body shape with gynaecomastia in adolescence, female distribution of body hair; enter puberty but sterile (adequate quantities of sperm not produced), hypogonadism (testes < 2 cm), upper to lower body segment ratio is low (limbs are elongated but not tall), breast cancer approaches frequency in female population, scoliosis, emphysema, diabetes mellitus, osteoporosis, varicose veins	usually presents due to sterility, suspicions confirmed by chromosomal analysis	same as normal adult population; testosterone treatment by long-term implants—improves sperm production and body hair
Turner syndrome; incidence 1 in 2500 liveborn females	female XO (45 chromosomes); female with a single X chromosome; may be deletion of Xp isochromosome (has two long arms but no short arm and other defects affecting Xp)	lymphoedema of neonate (cystic hygroma and swollen extremities), short stature, loose skin at neck (webbing), cubitus valgus (large carrying angle), short fingers and toes (especially fourth metatarsal), frail nails, many naevi, gastrointestinal bleeding, widely spaced nipples, no secondary sexual characteristics, sterile (gonads degenerate to connective tissue streaks at birth), congenital heart disease (20%), unexplained hypertension (27%), kidney malformations, thyroiditis, Crohn's disease, occult aneurysms of cerebral arteries	rarely detected on fetal ultrasound; usually presents with primary amenorrhoea or decreased growth; clinical suspicion is confirmed by chromosomal analysis	this syndrome has only mild mental retardation; life expectancy is below normal; administration of hormones at an appropriate age allows entry into puberty

Fig. 8.3 Features of some sex chromosome abnormalities.

normal body proportions. Although often asymptomatic, there may be subtle motor incoordination and behaviour problems, with aggression in childhood. Some increase in criminal behaviour is seen among XYY adults, but the vast majority do not fall foul of the law.

XX male

Y sequences are transferred to the X chromosome, with an incidence of 1 in 20 000 males. These males have a similar appearance to males with Klinefelter's syndrome, but:

- Are sterile.
- Show no skeletal disproportion.
- Have a normal IQ.

XX males usually present at the infertility clinic or when a prenatally predicted female appears to be male.

Confirmation is by banding studies, DNA analysis and in-situ hybridization, which identify Y-specific sequences.

Structural chromosomal abnormalities

These contiguous gene disorders are diagnosed with the light microscope by high-resolution banding. Deletion must involve at least three mega base pairs to be detected by this technique. It is important to find out whether the deletion has resulted *de novo* in the proband or from a balanced translocation in the parents. Recurrence is:

- Negligible with *de novo* mutations.
- Considerable with a balanced translocation.

Fig. 8.4 shows the features of some structural chromosomal disorders.

Features of some structural chromosome abnormalities		
Disorder	**Aetiology**	**Features**
Prader–Willi syndrome and Angelman syndrome; incidence 1 in 25 000 live births	both result from deletion in the same region on 15q11–13; syndromes differ due to genomic imprinting, so depend on which parent the deleted gene is inherited from—Prader–Willi syndrome results from inheritance of the deletion from the father (so only have maternal contribution to the critical area), Angelman syndrome results from inheritance of the deletion from the mother; uniparental disomy can result in these syndromes but does not involve deletions	Prader–Willi syndrome—neonatal hypotonia, initial feeding difficulties, obesity of face, trunk, and limbs (after first year of life), prominent forehead, almond-shaped eyes, triangular upper lips, IQ 20–80, short stature, small hands and feet, hypoplasia of external genitalia, tendency to diabetes mellitus. Angelman (happy puppet syndrome)—hypertonia, atoxic gait, characteristic arm posture, prominent jaw, deep set eyes, happy appearance, laughter, absent speech, mental retardation
Wolf–Hirschorn syndrome	partial deletion of the short arm of chromosome 4 (4p16.1); male to female ratio is 3:4	'Greek helmet' shaped head, cleft lip and palate, abnormal low-set ears, large beaked nose, hypertelorism (widely spaced eyes), epicanthic folds, microcephaly and mental retardation, failure to thrive, heart defects, convulsions, hypospadias
cri du chat syndrome	deletion of region on 5p15.2 or the whole short arm of chromosome 5	round face (in adults the face elongates), cat-like cry (*cri du chat*), hypertelorism, epicanthic folds, strabismus, low-set ears, low birth weight, mental retardation (variable degree), appear normal at birth

Fig. 8.4 Features of some structural chromosome abnormalities.

○ **Give examples of the major chromosomal disorders and describe their salient features.**

TRINUCLEOTIDE REPEAT DISORDERS

Introduction

Trinucleotide repeat expansions were first recognized as a mechanism for human disease in 1991 with the discovery of the expanded CGG triplet repeat that causes fragile X syndrome. Since then, nine more diseases have been associated with repeat expansions. Here the trinucleotide repeat disorders are described and their genetic aspects explained. A summary of the genetics of the trinucleotide repeat disorders is provided in Fig. 8.5.

Fragile X syndrome

The incidence of fragile X syndrome is 1 in 2250 males. It is X-linked, but one-third of carrier females have mild learning difficulties. One-fifth of affected males inheriting the defect are normal, but may pass the disease onto their grandsons. This is called Sherman's paradox, where the grandsons of 20% of males (carrying the FRAXA mutation, who are phenotypically normal), exhibit the full clinical phenotype. Therefore risk of mental retardation depends on the generation. Fragile X syndrome is the commonest inherited cause of learning difficulties.

Fragile X syndrome is caused by a triplet repeat expansion at Xq27.3; this is accompanied by a visible gap in the chromatin, which can be detected on metaphase chromosomes under certain cell culture conditions. The disorder is caused by an unstable expansion of a CGG trinucleotide in the 5'UTR (untranslated region) of the *FMR1* (fragile X mental retardation) gene. The defect is thought to cause hypermethylation of the *FMR1* gene, which shuts down its expression. FMR1 may regulate gene expression in the nervous system.

Clinical features, diagnosis, and prognosis

The clinical features of fragile X syndrome are:
- Male sex.
- Moderate learning difficulties (IQ 20–80).
- Macrocephaly.
- Macro-orchidism (usually post-puberty).
- Characteristic facies with a long face, prominent jaw, high forehead, and large everted ears.

Prenatal diagnosis can now be performed using DNA analysis. Males carrying the full mutation have either:
- A single larger band.
- A smear representing somatic instability.

	FRAX	HD	MD	SBMA	SCA-1	DRPLA
triplet repeat	CGG	CAG	CTG	CAG	CAG	CAG
position	Xq27.3	4p16.3	19q13.3	Xq11.12	6p22–23	12
increased repeat associated with greater disease severity?	no	yes	yes	yes	yes	yes
inheritance	X-linked	AD	AD	X-linked	AD	AD
severe juvenille onset?	no	yes	yes	no	yes	yes
anticipation?	no, but there is expansion in NTMs	yes	yes	no	yes	yes
most likely stage of repeat expansion	early embryogenesis	greatest instability during spermatogenesis	early embryogenesis	spermatogenesis	spermatogenesis	not known

Genetics of the trinucleotide repeat disorders

Fig. 8.5 Summary of the genetics of the trinucleotide repeat disorders. (FRAX, fragile X syndrome; HD, Huntington's disease; SBMA, spinobulbar muscular atrophy; SCA-1, spinocerebellar atrophy type 1. MD, myotonic dystrophy; DRPLA, dentatorubral-pallidoluysian atrophy.)

Individuals carrying a premutation have an intermediate sized band.

A normal life span can be expected, but lifestyle will be somewhat restricted because of the learning difficulties.

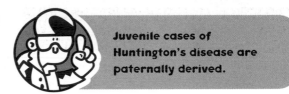

Juvenile cases of Huntington's disease are paternally derived.

Huntington's disease

The incidence of Huntington's disease is 1 in 10 000 Northern Europeans. It shows true autosomal dominance— homozygotes are no more severely affected than heterozygotes. The onset is usually in the fourth or fifth decades with increasing chorea and behavioural disturbances.

Juvenile onset of Huntington's disease is rare. It is associated with a severe form of the disease and early death. The severity of the disease is related to the size of the triplet repeat expansion. Repeat expansion seems to occur most frequently during spermatogenesis. Expansion is stable in maternal transmission.

The triplet repeat expansion, CAG, in the Huntingtin gene on 4p16.3 gives the gene product an expansion in the polyglutamine tract, that alters the function of the proteins. There is no reduction in the amount of transcript, but the triplet expansion alters the protein function—it may cause toxic accumulation of the gene product in the neuronal cells. The normal gene has 10–29 copies of the CAG repeat. In Huntington's disease there can be up to 120 copies (but usually there are 40–55).

Clinical features, diagnosis, and prognosis

The symptoms of Huntington's disease are associated with changes in the caudate nucleus due to loss of neurons that connect to the caudate nucleus from their origin in the corpus striatum. On magnetic resonance imaging (MRI) the neuronal loss is seen as flattening of the frontal horns of the lateral ventricles. The clinical features are:

- Personality changes.
- Psychiatric disorders such as severe depression.
- Progressive chorea.
- Dystonia.
- Dementia.

Diagnosis is by genetic testing, usually restriction fragment analysis or polymerase chain reaction (PCR).

The prognosis is poor, with death within 15–20 years of disease onset.

Myotonic dystrophy

The incidence of myotonic dystrophy is 1 in 8000. It is an autosomal dominant disorder with pronounced anticipation (i.e. increasing disease severity through generations). There are three forms with differing ages of onset:

- Mild—there is no muscle involvement and cataracts develop in middle or old age; the diagnosis is usually made because of family history of myotonic dystrophy.
- Moderate—myotonia and muscle weakness develop in adolescence or early adult life.
- Severe—this is characterized by congenital muscular hyperplasia, mental retardation, and a high neonatal mortality. The survivors develop the adult form of myotonic dystrophy before puberty.

Myotonic dystrophy is thought to be a result of a faulty kinase enzyme, dystrophica myotonica kinase (DM kinase), which occurs at neuromuscular junctions. Triplet repeat expansion of CTG occurs on chromosome 19q13.3 at the 3' end of the DM kinase gene. There tend to be:

- 50–99 repeats in mild disease.
- 100–1000 repeats in moderate disease.
- 1000–2000 repeats in severe disease.

Expansion appears to occur most readily after maternal transmission and occurs during early embryogenesis, but expansion or reduction can occur during transmission.

Clinical features, diagnosis, and prognosis

The clinical features of myotonic dystrophy are:

- Myotonia.
- Progressive muscle weakness and wasting.
- Associated symptoms of cardiac conduction defects, smooth muscle involvement, hypersomnia, cataracts, and an abnormal glucose response.
- In males, premature balding and testicular atrophy.

Diagnosis is based on the family history or molecular techniques.

157

Spinobulbar muscular atrophy (SBMA)

This neurodegenerative disorder is considerably less common than Huntington's disease, with an incidence of approximately 1 in 50 000. It is X-linked and female carriers can have symptoms (muscle cramps). It is caused by a defect in the androgen receptor gene on Xq11–12. There are signs of androgen insensitivity.

There is a characteristic degeneration of spinal and bulbar motor neurons and this may be caused by an expansion of CAG triplet repeats at the 3′ end of the gene.

Shake hands with the patient—patients with myotonic dystrophy characteristically have trouble relaxing their grip and letting go of your hand. You can therefore make the diagnosis before you have spoken to the patient!

Clinical features, diagnosis, and prognosis
The clinical features are:
- Usually male.
- Progressive muscle weakness and atrophy.
- Features of androgen insensitivity (i.e. gynaecomastia and reduced fertility).

The diagnosis is made by genetic analysis, usually PCR.

Spinocerebellar atrophy type 1 (SCA-1)

The onset of SCA-1 is usually in the third to fourth decade and the disease progresses to cause death due to bulbar dysfunction 10–20 years after the onset. There have been some juvenile cases, suggesting there may be anticipation. It is autosomal dominant and mapped to 6p22–23. There is a progressive neuronal loss in the cerebellum, brainstem, and spinocerebellar tracts.

Clinical features, diagnosis, and prognosis
The clinical features are:
- Ataxia.
- Dysarthria.
- Ophthalmoparesis.
- Variable degrees of muscle wasting.
- Neuropathy.

The prognosis is poor, with progression to death within 20 years of disease onset.

Dentatorubral-pallidoluysian atrophy (DRPLA)

DRPLA is an autosomal dominant condition. Familial cases have been found mainly in Japan, with a few sporadic cases in other countries. It is a progressive neurodegenerative disorder characterized by loss of neurons in the dentate nucleus, rubrum, globus pallidum, and Luys body. It is associated with a triplet repeat expansion on chromosome 12.

Clinical features, diagnosis, and prognosis
DRPLA causes a variety of symptoms including:
- Myoclonic epilepsy
- Choreiform movements.
- Cerebellar ataxia.
- Dementia.

The diagnosis is often based on a family history; recently, some families in Europe have been detected by molecular techniques.

Describe the basic pathology and clinical features of:
- Fragile X syndrome.
- Huntington's disease.
- Myotonic dystrophy.
- SBMA.
- SCA-1.
- DRPLA.

SINGLE GENE DISORDERS

Introduction
This section is a directory of the more important single gene disorders. Single gene disorders affect 1% of the population. The inheritance is mendelian, with mitochondrial inheritance being included for completeness.

Autosomal dominant inheritance
Fig. 8.6 summarizes the features of the following examples of autosomal dominant inherited disorders:

- Achondroplasia.
- Acute intermittent porphyria.
- Gilles de la Tourette's syndrome.
- Familial hypercholesterolaemia.
- Marfan syndrome.
- von Willebrand's disease.

A	Autosomal dominant disorders and their features		
Disorder	**Aetiology**	**Symptoms**	**Diagnosis, prognosis, and treatment**
achondroplasia; prevalence 1 in 10 000	mutation of the FGF receptor encoded on chromosome 3; causes decreased growth of cartilaginous bone; membranous bone is unaffected; 80% new mutation rate (i.e. 80% of cases are due to a mutation arising *de novo* in that individual, not inherited); increased incidence with paternal age; same gene with a different mutation causes a different phenotype (e.g. thanatophoric dwarfism, which is more severe, and hypochondroplasia, which is less severe)	large head, prominent forehead, short limbs, normal trunk size, lumbar lordosis	normal IQ and life expectancy
acute intermittent porphyria	mutation in porphobilinogen deaminase on chromosome 11; 80% are asymptomatic; environmental factors (e.g. drugs, alcohol, infection, or starvation) may trigger an attack	colicky abdominal pain, vomiting, constipation, fever, peripheral neuritis (may cause respiratory paralysis), psychosis	diagnosis: erythrocyte porphobilinogen deaminase assay; treatment—avoid environmental triggers and treat acute attacks with sedation, pain relief, electrolyte balance, carbohydrate, anticonvulsant, antiemetic, propanolol and physiotherapy; prognosis—fatal in 5%
Gilles de la Tourette syndrome; prevalence 1 in 2000	unknown	motor and verbal tics (often obscene or animal noises), obsessive–compulsive behaviour, attention deficit, learning difficulties	diagnosis—tics for over 1 year; treatment—haloperidol or clonidine; prognosis—often improves with age
familial hyper-cholesterolaemia	mutation in LDL receptor gene on chromosome 19	at 30–40 years—xanthoma, xanthelasma, corneal arcus, ischaemic heart disease	diagnosis—family history, increased fasting LDL and cholesterol; definitive diagnosis by DNA pedigree analysis of RFLPs or specific mutations

B	Aetiology, symptoms and treatment of Marfan syndrome and von Willebrand's disease		
Disorder	**Aetiology**	**Symptoms**	**Diagnosis, prognosis, and treatment**
Marfan syndrome	mutation in gene coding for connective tissue factors	arachnodactyly (long spidery limbs and fingers); armspan > height; upper to lower segment ratio ↓; high-arched palate, lens dislocation, aortic incompetence	diagnosis—clinical, combined with ECG; treatment—β blockers may slow aortic dilatation; life expectancy 40–50 years due to CVS complications
von Willebrand's disease	deficiency of von Willebrand's factor (vWF) which adheres platelets and binds to factor VIII, preventing its breakdown	haemorrhage from mucosal sites and postoperatively	diagnosis—vWF low, factor VIII activity low, prolonged bleeding time, normal platelet count and whole-blood clotting time; treatment—vasopressin, factor VIII, cryoprecipitate

Fig. 8.6 (A) Features of examples of autosomal dominant disorders. (LDL, low-density lipoproteins; RFLPs, restriction fragment length polymorphisms.) (B) Marfan syndrome and von Willebrand's disease. (AFP, α-fetoprotein; CVS, cardiovascular system; ECG, electrocardiogram; HCG, human chorionic gonadotrophin.)

Autosomal recessive inheritance

Fig. 8.7 summarizes the features of the following examples of autosomal recessive disorders:

- α Thalassaemia.
- β Thalassaemia.
- Congenital adrenal hyperplasia.
- Cystic fibrosis.
- Friedreich's ataxia.
- Gaucher's disease.
- Haemochromatosis.
- Phenylketonuria.
- Sickle cell disease.
- Tay–Sachs disease.

X-linked recessive inheritance

Fig. 8.8 summarizes the features of the following examples of X-linked recessive disorders:

- Adrenoleucodystrophy.
- Duchenne muscular dystrophy.
- Becker muscular dystrophy.
- Fabry's disease.
- Glucose-6-phosphate dehydrogenase (G6PD) deficiency
- Haemophilia A.
- Haemophila B (Christmas disease).
- Lesch–Nyhan syndrome.

Autosomal recessive disorders and their features			
Disorder	**Aetiology**	**Symptoms**	**Diagnosis, prognosis, and treatment**
Gaucher's disease; incidence 1 in 25 000; carriers 1 in 15 Ashkenazi Jews	mutation in β glucosidase, encoded on chromosome 1; causes glucocerebrosidase accumulation	type I (adult)—no neurological features, onset 2–70 years, bone pain, splenomegaly; type II (infantile)—marked neurological symptoms, onset 1–2 months, hepatosplenomegaly, death by 2 years of age; type III (juvenile)—neurological symptoms present, onset at 5 years	diagnosis—biochemical assay of β glucosidase activity; treatment—enzyme replacement therapy, bone marrow transplant (only if severe) and gene therapy in the future; prognosis—assay does not predict prognosis, which depends on phenotype I, II, or III
haemochromatosis	primary is inherited via a gene on chromosome 6; secondary is caused by another disease or transfusion	excess iron accumulates in tissues, especially liver, causing cirrhosis, cardiomyopathy, and diabetes mellitus	diagnosis—high transferrin saturation, high serum iron, high serum ferritin; liver biopsy is definitive; treatment—venesection.
phenylketonuria	mutation of phenylalanine hydroxylase encoded on chromosome 12	decreased IQ, fair hair, fits, eczema, musty urine; untreated affected females have malformed offspring	treatment—diet low in phenylalanine, with tyrosine supplements for entire life; diagnosis—elevated blood or urine phenylalanine; mandatory test in all neonates by Guthrie heel prick test
sickle cell disease	point mutation Glu-6 to Val on position 6 of β globin gene encoded on chromosome 11p (HbA to HbS); distorted sickle-shaped cells by polymerization of deoxygenated HbS; sickle cells can block vessels or haemolyse; electrophoresis—majority HbS, some HbA2, persistence of HbF; common in Africans	homozygotes (SS)—haemolytic anaemia, infarction (e.g. hand and foot syndrome), splenomegaly early, then splenic infarction after more than 10 years, respiratory infections, osteomyelitis (especially *Salmonella*), crises (painful bone marrow aplasia, sequestration or haemolytic) often triggered by infections; heterozygote (AS); heterozygote has an advantage against cerebral malaria; hypoxia may precipitate an occlusive crisis	diagnosis—prenatal diagnosis by direct assay involves PCR amplification of the relevant β globin region, followed by digestion with a restriction enzyme as *Mst*II mustine restriction site lost; carrier detection by haematological assay (e.g Hb electrophoresis); treatment—pneumococcal vaccine and support during crises, prognosis—decreased life expectancy in HbSS
Tay–Sachs disease; carrier 1 in 250 in general population; 1 in 25 in Ashkenazi Jews	lysosomal storage disorder; mutation in hexaminidase A α chain encoded on chromosome 15 causes ganglioside GM2 accumulation	progressive neurological abnormalities begin in late infancy; cherry red macular spot in 90% (not pathognomonic); decreased serum β N-acetyl hexosaminidase activity; death at 3–4 years of age	diagnosis—carrier screening in Jewish population; carrier detection by decreased hexosaminidase levels on assay; prenatal diagnosis by assay on fetal samples; treatment—no specific treatment, just supportive

Fig. 8.7 Features of examples of autosomal recessive disorders. (ACTH, adrenocorticotrophic hormone; FBC, full blood count; HBA, haemoglobin A; HbF, haemoglobin F; MCV, mean red cell volume; MCHC, mean red cell haemoglobin concentration; PCR, polymerase chain reaction.)

Autosomal recessive disorders and their features *(cont.)*			
Disorder	**Aetiology**	**Symptoms**	**Diagnosis, prognosis, and treatment**
α thalassaemia	the fetus normally has HbF (α_2,γ_2); normal adults have 95% HbA (α_2,β_2) and a small amount of HbA2 (α_2,δ_2); mutation occurs in the two α globin genes encoded on chromosome 16p; each person has two chromosome 16s, so four α globin genes ($\alpha\alpha$, $\alpha\alpha$); severity depends on the number of functional α genes; this disorder is more common in Black populations	α thalassamia type I homozygotes (– –/– –) have no functional α globin genes, resulting in hydrops fetalis; in haemoglobin H disease (– –/– α) there is a single α globin gene and a good prognosis; the following have absence of one or two genes, resulting in mild anaemia—α thalassaemia type 2 homozygote (– α/– α), α thalassaemia type γ heterozygote (– –/$\alpha\alpha$), α thalassaemia type 2 heterozygote (–α/$\alpha\alpha$)	diagnosis—Hb electrophoresis, FBC, MCV; α thalassaemia type I homozygote—80% haemoglobin Barts (four γ chains), persistent fetal haemoglobin; haemoglobin H disease —some haemoglobin Barts, 5–30% HbH (four β chains), reduced MCHC and MCV; treatment—transfusion, iron chelation, folate, ascorbic acid, and splenectomy in hypersplenism
β thalassaemia	mutation in β globin gene encoded on 11p; common in Mediterranean populations, Chinese, Indians and American Blacks	severe chronic haemolytic anaemia; iron overload (despite chelation) causes endocrine, liver, and heart failure	diagnosis and treatment—as in α thalassaemia; β thalassaemia major —blood film (hypochromic microcytic cells and target cells), HbF increases, HbA2 variable, HbA absent; β thalassaemia minor—HbA2 > 3.5%, mild anaemia and decreased MCV; moderate mutational heterogeneity but each population has a prevalent set of mutations; mutations are detected by using the indirect method of a bank of related assays (the reverse dot-blot method); prenatal diagnosis is available; prognosis— minor has good prognosis, major results in death within 1 year if not treated with transfusions; with transfusions death occurs at 20–40 years of age due to iron overload
congenital adrenal hyperplasia	mutation in 21-hydroxylase gene on chromosome 6 which produces aldosterone and cortisone; absence of enzyme causes precursor conversion into testosterone	masculinization of female genitalia, precocious puberty in male, salt-losing crises may occur owing to deficiency of mineralocorticoid (mainly aldosterone)	diagnosis—low cortisol and aldosterone, high ACTH levels (no negative feedback)
cystic fibrosis; incidence 1 in 2000 Caucasians; carrier rate is 1 in 22 of UK population	gene on 7q31 encodes chloride channel transmembrane conductance regulator; defective regulation of chloride transport results in accumulation of thick viscid secretions in pancreas, respiratory, gastrointestinal, and genitourinary tracts; 68% of CF mutations are deletion of phenylalanine at codon 508 (Δ508)	chronic obstructive airways disease, shortness of breath, pancreatic insufficiency, failure to thrive, malabsorption, meconium ileus; male infertility (some mild forms present with this), fatal heat prostration	diagnosis—sweat test [Na$^+$] + [Cl$^-$] > 70 mM; prenatal diagnosis—Brock test (microvillar enzymes in amniotic fluid); population screening not undertaken as lack of absolute association between particular mutations and severity, cannot tell parents how severely affected the child may be, and life expectancy is into the 40s; treatment—pancreatic enzyme supplements, diet, physiotherapy clears lungs, inhalers, nebulizers, antibiotics for infections, heart/lung transplant and gene therapy (currently trials with nasal spray); prognosis— until recently death in infancy or childhood, now many live into 40s.
Friedreich's ataxia	gene located on 7q, encodes 'fraxitin'; spinocerebellar degeneration with cerebellar ataxia and degeneration of posterior columns and cortico– spinal and spinocerebellar tract	at 6–8 years develop ataxia, pigeon chest, loss of deep tendon reflexes in legs, extensor plantars; need wheelchair in 20s	prognosis—life expectancy into 50th year of life

Fig. 8.7 *cont.*

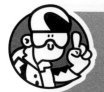

Always read all questions carefully. For example, creatine and creatinine are similar but are not the same molecule—you can get trapped if you do not pay attention!

X-linked dominant inheritance
Vitamin D-resistant rickets
This disorder of defective tubular phosphate reabsorption results in growth retardation and rickets. Treatment is with vitamin D and phosphate.

Single gene disorders with more than one mode of inheritance
Fig. 8.9 summarizes the features of examples of single

X-linked recessive disorders and their features			
Disorder	**Aetiology**	**Symptoms**	**Diagnosis, prognosis, and treatment**
glucose-6-phosphate dehydrogenase (G6PD) deficiency	G6PD enzyme defect on Xq28; erythrocytes susceptible to oxidative damage, which is often precipitated by drugs, illness, or fava beans	haemolytic anaemia; variable phenotype, most severe resulting in neonatal jaundice	diagnosis—enzyme assay; treatment includes avoiding precipitating factors
haemophilia A; incidence 1 in 5000 liveborn males	mutation in factor VIII locus, on Xq28; gene product is involved in intrinsic blood coagulation pathway.	recurrent haemorrhage into soft tissues and joints when levels less than 30% (severity varies)	diagnosis—prenatal diagnosis by fetal sampling and DNA analysis, direct and definitive; carrier detection by pedigree studies using RFLPs; less accurate carrier detection possible by factor VIII coagulation (but result may be spuriously normal due to random X inactivation); treatment—administer coagulation factor; risk of producing inhibitor complication where antibodies are produced against 'foreign therapeutic coagulation factors'—this complication may arise if the mutation results in no factor VIII being produced so the immune system is not primed; prognosis—blood transfusions during the 1980s inadvertently transmitted bloodborne viruses (e.g. HIV, hepatitis B, C, and D), which have decreased the life expectancy of many patients transfused over this period, so now all factor VIII is screened and tested to eliminate HIV and hepatitis B and C
haemophilia B (Christmas disease); incidence 1 in 30 000 liveborn males	mutation of factor IX gene on Xq27.1; factor IX is involved in the coagulation cascade	haemorrhage usually less severe than in haemophilia A	diagnosis—highly heterogenous mutation, so needs direct diagnosis by sequencing the mutation in the family under investigation, as in haemophilia A; treatment—administer coagulation factor; risk of inhibitor complication but less than for haemophilia A; prognosis—decreased life expectancy in those that have acquired bloodborne infections through transfusion as HIV rarely contaminated factor IX preparation
Lesch–Nyhan syndrome	disorder of purine synthesis causing hyperuricaemia and reduced erythrocyte hypoxanthine–guanine phosphoribosyltransferase	spasticity, mental retardation, self-harm, renal stones, gouty arthritis	diagnosis—enzyme assay of HPRT; treatment—allopurinol (does not affect neurological signs)
adreno-leucodystrophy	type 3 peroxisomal disorder, due to a single enzyme defect; enzyme affected is involved in β oxidation	onset is at 4–5 years, with behavioural, visual, and neurological abnormalities	diagnosis—first made by measuring metabolites, then confirmed by enzyme assay

Fig. 8.8 Features of examples of X-linked recessive disorders. (EMG, electromyography; RFLPs, restriction fragment length polymorphisms).

gene disorders with more than one mode of inheritance.

Mitochondrial inheritance

The phenotype is related to the severity of oxidative phosphorylation defect, and the organ's dependence on ATP production. The severity of the disorder in any individual increases with age due to the natural decline of oxidative enzymes and accumulation of mutations in mitochondrial DNA.

Inheritance is sporadic, maternal, or mendelian. Mendelian inheritance is due to a nuclear gene, which interacts with mitochondrial function.

Clinical features and diagnosis

Symptoms have an early onset, with a rapid progression of unexplained symptoms in unrelated organs, for example:

- Metabolic ketoacidotic coma.
- Hepatic failure.
- Bone marrow symptoms.
- Cardiac involvement.
- Renal tubular involvement.
- Gastrointestinal symptoms (failure to thrive, diarrhoea).
- Endocrine pancreas (diabetes mellitus).
- Dwarfism.
- Skin rashes.
- Hypotonia.
- Leber's optic atrophy.
- Muscle weakness with myopathy.

Diagnosis is by detection of increased (lactate) accumulation:

- The lactate:pyruvate ratio is increased.
- Cerebrospinal fluid (CSF) (lactate) is increased.
- Ketone bodies are increased.

X-linked recessive disorders and their features (cont.)			
Disorder	Aetiology	Symptoms	Diagnosis, prognosis, and treatment
Duchenne muscular dystrophy (DMD); incidence 1 in 3500 liveborn males	most common severe X-linked disease; mutation in Xp21 coding for cytoskeletal protein dystrophin, causes protein to lose its C-terminal proteins; one-third are new mutations; 2–3 Mb, largest known gene, dystrophin prevents the muscle from tearing during contraction and prevents degeneration of muscle fibres; fibre appearance—variation in fibre size, eosinophilic fibres (with intracellular calcium), increased connective tissue between fibres and lipid droplet accumulations	30% have decreased IQ; electroretinopathy (form of night blindness), increased phospho-fructokinase; newborn appears normal; at 3–4 years of age there is difficulty rising from sitting (Gower's manoeuvre—climbing up legs), pseudohypertrophy of calf muscles, deltoid, scapula, and quadriceps (muscle replaced by fat and connective tissue) and cardiomyopathy; at 6 years of age ambulation is difficult (require callipers), symmetrical wasting; at 12 years of age most are wheelchair bound and have scoliosis; die at 17–20 years of age due to respiratory insufficiency	diagnosis—creatine kinase grossly elevated; EMG myopathic; DNA analysis—many mutations possible, need to isolate family-specific mutation and set up an assay for clinical diagnosis (60% are deletions or duplications, 40% are point mutations); stain for dystrophin on muscle biopsy—absent; carrier detection by creatine kinase assay and definitive DNA analysis (risks only lowered to 5–10% due to germline mosaicism); treatment— physiotherapy, prednisolone (a catabolic steroid which helps to preserve muscle strength), minimal bed rest when ill or may never walk again; ambulation aids—callipers, percutaneous tenotomy, foot orthosis, etc; early spinal fusion; monitor heart (protected to a degree by lack of mobility; do not fuse spine if severe cardiomyopathy as anaesthetics cannot be given; nasal ventilation at night (decreases somnolence); gene therapy awaited; prognosis—death in early 20s
Becker muscular dystrophy; incidence 1 in 30 000 liveborn males	mutation in Xp21 gene causes the middle of the dystrophin protein to be absent, affecting dystrophin packaging	at 16 years of age wheelchair bound; some have cardiomyopathy; there is an intermediate phenotype to DMD with loss of ambulation at 12–16 years of age	diagnosis—creatine kinase increased, EMG myopathic; DNA deletion screen; stain for dystrophin on muscle biopsy—present; ECG and echocardiogram show cardiomyopathy; treatment—prednisolone; prognosis—near-normal life expectancy
Fabry's disease	deficiency of galactosidase A, causes accumulation of ceramide in skin, kidneys, and cardiovascular system	angiokeratoma; cardiovascular system—infarction, angina, valve lesions, cardiomyopathy	prognosis—live into 50s

Fig. 8.8 cont.

Single gene disorders with more than one mode of inheritance			
Disorder	**Aetiology**	**Symptoms**	**Diagnosis, prognosis, and treatment**
Alport's syndrome; carrier frequency 1 in 5000	X-linked or autosomal recessive glomerulonephritis; associated with sensorineural deafness and eye lesions; genes affected each code for different α chains of type IV collagen— chains of type IV collagen— α_1 (COL4A1) on chromosome 13, α_2 (COL4A2) on chromosome 13, α_3 (COL4A3) on chromosome 2, α_4 (COL4A4) on chromosome 2, α_5 (COL4A5) on Xq22; type IV collagen is the major structural protein in the basement membrane; type COL4A5 is important in the basement membrane of glomeruli, lens, and organ of Corti	by 5 years of age—microscopic haematuria; by 10 years—high-tone deafness; mid-teens—increased blood pressure; by 20 years—increased plasma creatinine; by 25 years—end-stage renal failure; associated with leiomyomatosis; females have a more variable clinical course due to random X inactivation	renal failure
Charcot–Marie–Tooth syndrome (peroneal muscular atrophy)	also known as hereditary motor and sensory neuropathy type I; inheritance usually AD (chromosome 17) but can be AR or X-linked dominant; genetically determined polyneuropathies, classified according to inheritance	progressive from puberty— foot drop, leg weakness, 'inverted champagne bottle' legs (ankles are the corks), general limb weakness, diminished sensation and reflexes	diagnosis—nerve biopsy shows demyelination
Ehlers–Danlos syndrome	abnormal collagen affects skin, joints, and vasculature; inheritance usually AD but may be AR or X-linked	lax skin, hypermobile joints, scoliosis, purpura (skin bruising), bleeding of internal organs, fragile eyes	prognosis—decreased if vasculature is affected
mucopoly-saccharidoses; incidence 7 in 100 000 live births	lysosomal storage disorders; uronic acid alternates with an amino sugar in a mucopolysaccharide; degradation occurs in a stepwise manner, with any deficient enzyme resulting in a disease; AR inheritance except for the following X-linked diseases (e.g. Hurler syndrome, Sanfilippo syndrome, Hunter syndrome)	progressive neurological degeneration, hepato/splenomegaly, skeletal dysplasia, short stature, bone pain, coarse facies, eyes—cherry red spots, corneal clouding	diagnosis—biochemical identification of mucopolysaccharides in urine and amniotic fluid
polycystic kidney disease; incidence AD 1 in 1000, AR 1 in 40 000; carrier frequency 1 in 100	primary polycystic kidney disease (PKD) is either adult (AD) or infantile (AR); secondary PKD may have no genetic link (e.g. due to obstructive anomalies *in utero*); AD PKD type 1 due to mutation on chromosome 16; type II mutation unknown; AR PKD—gene affected is on chromosome 6, causing disease with four distinct levels of severity	normally fatal in infants; adult type symptoms—loin pain, renal colic, hypertension, haematuria (blood in urine), urinary tract infection, uraemia	AD PKD type II has a more benign course than type I; AR PKD—perinatal rapidly die at birth, neonatal (onset neonatal) die by 3 months; infantile (onset in first 6 months)—liver cysts prominent; juvenile (onset at 1–5 years of age)—severe liver involvement
retinitis pigmentosa	AD, AR, or X-linked variants; macrophages around retinal vessels accumulate melanin from the choroid	progressive night blindness and tunnel vision	diagnosis—visualize retinal pigment particles; prognosis—progressive blindness
severe combined immuno-deficiency	many AR and X-linked variants; adenosine deficiency; purine nucleoside phosphorylase deficiency	recurrent viral, fungal, and bacterial infections; failure to thrive	treatment—traditionally by marrow transplant; first disease to be treated by gene therapy (1990); prognosis—death in infancy if untreated

Fig. 8.9 Features of examples of single gene disorders with more than one mode of inheritance. (AD, autosomal dominant; AR, autosomal recessive; Col4 A×, collagen type IV of × type α chain.

Syndromes

The syndromes are:

- MELAS—encephalopathy, stroke, lactic acidosis.
- MERAF—epilepsy, cardiomyopathy, encephalopathy.
- Leber's optic atrophy (worse in smokers).
- Kearns'—neurological.
- Pearson's—bone marrow failure, pancreatic symptoms; survivors develop Kearns' syndrome.
- Cox deficiency—encephalopathy, myopathy, Fanconi syndrome, liver failure.

No treatment is available. Prenatal diagnosis is available for affected mothers.

> Give examples of the major single gene disorders and describe their salient features.

GENETIC CANCER SYNDROMES

Overview

There are over 200 single disorders that have cancer as a recognizable complication. A large proportion of these are the result of the loss of one copy of a tumour suppressor gene. If a somatic event causes the loss of the remaining functioning allele (the 'second hit'—see Fig. 6.21), malignant progression is very likely. This phenomenon, in which a single functioning allele of the tumour suppressor is lost, is called loss of constitutional heterozygosity (LOCH).

Features suggestive of an inherited cancer susceptibility in a family

These are:

- Several close (first or second degree) relatives with a common cancer.
- Several close relatives with genetically associated cancers (e.g. breast and ovary, or bowel and endometrial).
- Two family members with the same rare cancer.

- An unusually early age of onset.
- Bilateral tumours in paired organs.
- Synchronous or successive tumours.
- Tumours in two different organ systems in one individual.

Some of the commoner genetic cancer syndromes are discussed below.

Ataxia telangiectasia

This is an autosomal recessive disorder that affects 1 in 50 000. The *ATM* gene involved has been mapped to 11q23. It is thought to be involved in p53-mediated cell cycle arrest and apoptosis—that is, loss of function of the gene results in:

- Loss of cell cycle arrest.
- Loss of programmed cell death in response to DNA damage.

The onset is usually in childhood with progressive cerebellar ataxia, recurrent infections, and oculocutaneous telangiectasias. It is caused by a DNA repair defect and involves failure to excise nucleotide bases damaged by γ radiation. These children have a raised serum α fetoprotein and have non-random chromosome rearrangements. Approximately 30% die of myeloproliferative disease before 9 years of age.

Familial breast cancer

This accounts for about 5% of breast cancer and often presents at an early age. Mutations in the *BRCA-1* gene on 17q and *BRCA-2* gene on 13q account for over 50% of these cases. Both mutations have highly penetrant autosomal dominant inheritance and are associated with specific cancers as follows:

- *BRCA-1* mutations are associated with breast and ovarian cancer, and also an excess of prostate and colon cancer.
- *BRCA-2* mutations are associated with breast, endometrial, renal, and bladder cancer. They are also associated with laryngeal carcinomas, lymphomas, and, occasionally, male breast cancer.

DNA testing is available for large families with breast cancer (e.g. 1% of Ashkenazi Jews have a 185delAG mutation in *BRCA-1*, which can be screened for).

Prophylactic bilateral mastectomies are sometimes considered following DNA analysis for women with a very strong family history.

Familial adenomatous polyposis coli

This is a rare autosomal dominant condition caused by a deletion in 5q21 resulting in a loss of function of the tumour suppressor gene, *APC*. This leads to the development of multiple benign adenomatous polyps of the large bowel (Fig. 8.10). A somatic mutation can result in the development of adenocarcinoma due to LOCH (see above).

The diagnosis is based on:

- Family history.
- The presence of multiple intestinal polyps from childhood.

There are also characteristic retinal changes in 80% of families.

There is a 90% risk of malignancy, and prophylactic whole-colon resection is often considered.

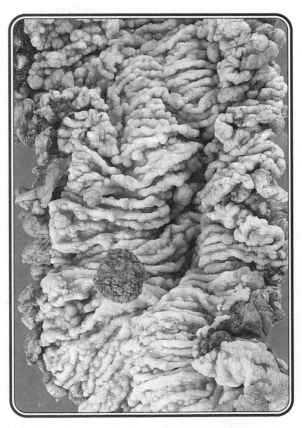

Fig. 8.10 Polyposis coli in large bowel. The multiple adenomatous polyps are clearly visible. (Courtesy of Dr A. Stevens and Professor J. Lowe.)

Fanconi syndrome

Fanconi's syndrome is inherited as an autosomal recessive trait with an incidence of 1 in 350 000. More than one gene is associated with the syndrome. There is a DNA repair defect resulting in sensitivity to agents causing interstrand crosslinks (e.g. alkylating agents).

The clinical features include:

- Pancytopenia.
- Skin pigmentation.
- Congenital malformations including radial limb defects.

Acute non-lymphocytic leukaemia develops in 5–10% of cases. Hepatocellular carcinoma and squamous cell carcinoma are also associated.

Li–Fraumeni syndrome

This is a rare autosomal dominant trait and is often due to mutation in the *p53* gene on 17p. It is commonly characterized by childhood cancers such as:

- Soft tissue sarcomas.
- Adrenal carcinomas.
- Brain tumours.

Later there is a high frequency of breast cancer, astrocytoma, and lung cancer. Direct mutation analysis is often possible, but of little benefit. The prognosis depends upon the number and sites of tumours.

Hereditary non-polyposis coli

This is an autosomal dominant trait in which there is familial clustering of early-onset colon cancer (70% proximal). The condition is associated with germ-line mutations in the DNA mismatch repair family of genes. Mutations in four genes—*hMSH2*, *hMLH1*, *hPMS1*, and *hPMS2*—have been identified so far. Relatives are recommended to have yearly colonoscopy from 20–25 years of age.

Multiple endocrine neoplasias (MEN)

These are subdivided into MEN I, IIa, and IIb. They are rare autosomal dominant conditions:

- MEN I has been associated with the loss of a tumour suppressor gene mapped to 11q13.
- MEN IIa and IIb are caused by mutations in the RET oncogene on chromosome 10.

The clinical features are as follows:

- MEN I is characterized by pituitary adenoma, hyperparathyroidism, and pancreatic adenomas (often gastrinomas, accounting for 50% of patients with Zollinger–Ellison syndrome).
- MEN IIa is characterized by phaeochromocytoma, medullary thyroid carcinoma, and hyperparathyroidism.
- MEN IIb is characterized by neuromas of the mucous membranes, phaeochromocytoma, megacolon, and medullary thyroid carcinoma (Fig. 8.11).

Prenatal diagnosis is now possible by direct mutation analysis and MEN IIa and IIb are monitored by yearly calcitonin assays from 5–30 years of age for early detection of medullary thyroid carcinoma.

Neurofibromatosis type I (von Recklinghausen's disease)

This has an incidence of 1 in 3000. It is an autosomal dominant condition in which there is a mutation in the tumour suppressor gene *NF1* on 17q. *NF1* is thought to be responsible for catalyzing the hydrolysis of 'Ras-GTP', an activated intracellular protein complex that brings about cell cycle progression. Loss of *NF1* causes accumulation of Ras-GTP resulting in an increased rate of cell turnover.

The condition has variable expression and is characterized by:

- *Café-au-lait* patches.
- Skin neurofibromas.
- Axillary freckling.
- Iris hamartomas.
- Spinal and autonomic neuromas.
- Phaeochromocytoma.

Complications include scoliosis, learning difficulties, and seizures. Approximately 4% of cases develop central nervous system (CNS) tumours and 3% develop other tumours. The role of ketotifen in the management of neurofibrosarcoma is under evaluation.

Neurofibromatosis type II

This is also autosomal dominant. It has an incidence of 1 in 35 000 due to a variety of mutations in the tumour

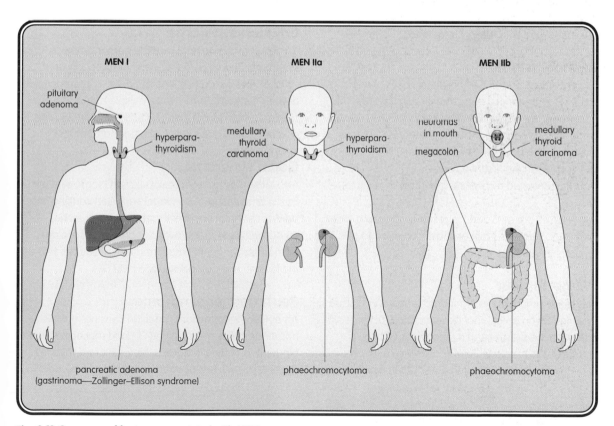

Fig. 8.11 Summary of features associated with MEN.

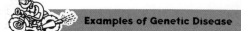

suppressor *NF2* on chromosome 22q. It is characterized by:
- Bilateral acoustic neuromas.
- Intracranial meningiomas.
- *Café-au-lait* patches.
- Lens opacities.
- CNS tumours.

Prenatal diagnosis is possible by direct and indirect DNA analysis and carriers can be offered screening with MRI and audiology.

Tuberous sclerosis
This is an autosomal dominant trait with loci on 9q (TSC1) and 16p (TSC2). It has an incidence of 1 in 10 000 and there are characteristic skin changes in early childhood including:
- White patches seen under ultraviolet light (Wood's lamp).
- A fibroangiomatous rash.

Intracranial calcification and periventricular hamartomas are seen on computerized tomography (CT); 90% of cases develop epilepsy and 60% of cases are associated with mental retardation.

Retinoblastoma
Bilateral cases and 15% of unilateral cases of this childhood tumour of the eye are inherited as an autosomal dominant trait due to a mutation in the *Rb* gene on chromosome 13q14 (see page 69). There is an incidence of 1 in 18 000. The onset:
- Is usually in the first two years.
- Is first detected by a white light reflex or a squint.

Some cases are detected by neonatal screening for a red reflex. Survivors have an increased risk of adult tumours in various organs.

Wilms' tumour
This renal tumour is mostly sporadic; however, 1% are inherited as an autosomal dominant trait. Diagnosis is based on the presence of a renal mass with characteristic histology. Some cases are associated with a microdeletion syndrome at 11p13 in which there is

aniridia and mental and growth retardation (WAGR). There is an increased risk of Wilms' tumour in Beckwith–Wiedermann syndrome.

Xeroderma pigmentosum
This has an incidence of 1 in 70 000. There are at least nine subgroups and these are characterized by:
- Defective DNA excision repair.
- Extreme ultraviolet light sensitivity.

Clinical features of xeroderma pigmentosum are:
- Progressive corneal and skin scarring on exposure to sunlight.
- Multiple skin cancers by 20 years of age.

von Hippel–Lindau disease
A rare condition mapped to 3p25–26, Affected individuals characteristically have multiple renal cysts and early onset of bilateral, multifocal renal carcinoma (clear cell carcinoma). CNS tumours are also associated. These tend to be haemangioblastomas, which are benign but associated with high morbidity.

Cowden syndrome
An autosomal dominant multiple hamartomatous syndrome. There is progressive macrocephaly in childhood with mild to moderate delay in psychomotor development. Adults develop multiple hamartomas. There is a high risk of thyroid, GI, breast, and ovarian cancers (which often develop in harmartomas).

Gorlin syndrome
Also known as naevoid basal cell carcinoma syndrome. This is an autosomal dominant condition causing a predisposition to basal cell carcinoma of the skin, medulloblastoma, and ovarian fibromas. There are associated congenital malformations including dental malformations, cleft palate, and bifid ribs.

Peutz Jegher syndrome
An autosomal dominant condition causing multiple hamartomatous polyps in the GIT and mucocutaneous pigmented lesions in the lips, face, and oral mucosa. There is a 2–3% risk of adenocarcinoma of the GIT.

Describe the genetic basis and general clinical features of:
- Ataxia telangiectasia.
- Familial breast cancer.
- Fanconi syndrome.
- Familial adenomatous polyposis coli.
- Hereditary non-polyposis coli.
- MEN I, IIa, and IIb.
- Neurofibromatosis type I and II.
- Tuberous sclerosis.
- Retinoblastoma.
- Wilms' tumour.
- Xeroderma pigmentosum.

CONGENITAL MALFORMATIONS

Definition

A malformation is a primary error of development. By definition all malformations must be congenital (present at birth), but for medicolegal purposes they are recorded as congenital only if they are detected within the first two weeks of life. The incidence percentage among newborns is:

- 14% have a single minor malformation.
- 3% have a single major malformation.
- 0.7% have multiple major malformations.

The aetiology percentage is:

- 60% are idiopathic.
- 20% are multifactorial.
- 7.5% are monogenic.
- 6% are chromosomal.
- 3% are due to maternal illness.
- 2% are due to congenital infection.
- 1.5% are due to drugs, X-rays, alcohol.

Maternal insulin-dependent diabetes mellitus is associated with:

- Congenital heart disease.
- Neural tube defect.
- Phocomelia (seal-shaped, fused lower limb).
- Sacral agenesis.

The risk is higher if the diabetes mellitus is poorly controlled.

Maternal epilepsy is associated with:
- Cleft lip.
- Congenital heart disease.

It is hard to ascertain whether the increase is related to the disease or the medication.

A number of congenital infections are known to cause multiple malformations (Fig. 8.12).

Congenital deformations

A deformation is a defect caused by abnormal compression of the fetus *in utero*. It is correctable and usually resolves completely in the neonatal period.

Congenital dislocation of the hip

Temporary clicking is a feature of 4–7 in 1000 live births; 1 in 1000 has a dislocation; 6♀:1♂. It is multifactorial, involving both genetic and environmental factors. It is commoner in populations where babies are swaddled (e.g. Eskimos, South Americans) and very rare in

Congenital infections causing multiple malformations are called the TORCH infections (T, toxoplasmosis; O, other (e.g. syphilis); R, rubella; C, cytomegalovirus; H, herpes).

populations where children are carried on backs with legs astride (e.g. Africans). There is an increased risk if there is a positive family history or breech birth, or if the infant has a neuromuscular disorder.

Diagnosis, management, and prognosis

All neonates are checked routinely by flexing the hips and knees and then gently abducting the thighs while lifting the greater trochanter forwards. If the hips are lax, a 'clunk' is felt. Management involves setting the pelvis in a 'frog' splint with hips abducted. The prognosis is very good if the deformity is detected early.

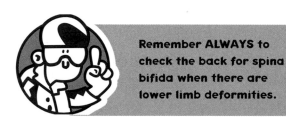

Remember ALWAYS to check the back for spina bifida when there are lower limb deformities.

Talipes equinovarus (club foot)

The incidence is 1.2 in 1000 live births; 3♂:1♀. It is related to the infant's position *in utero*. The risk increases 20-fold if a first degree relative is affected. Rarely there is an underlying neurological problem. The feet are plantarflexed and inverted. It is detected on routine neonatal check and is usually corrected by gentle manipulation and strapping during the first few weeks of life. Correction should be achieved within the first three months of life or surgical correction of bone deformity will be required later in childhood.

Limb defects (malformations, not deformations)

Two live births in every 1000 have a major limb malformation.

Polydactyly (extra digits)

This is seen in 1 in 2000 Caucasians. It may be a feature of:

Congenital infections			
Congenital infection	**Critical period during pregnancy**	**Malformations**	**Additional notes**
toxoplasmosis	12% risk at 6–17 weeks; 60% risk at 17–28 weeks	mental handicap, microcephaly, chorioretinitis	source of infection usually undercooked meat, or cat litter; maternal infection often asymptomatic; prophylactic treatment with spiromycin if infection suspected; rare in UK so mothers not screened
syphilis	8 months to term	congenital syphilis; may have stigmata such as collapsed nasal bridge	now rare in the developed countries; all pregnant women are screened at booking as congenital syphilis can be avoided by a simple course of penicillin taken by the mother
rubella	first 6 weeks	patent ductus arteriosus, microcephaly, mental handicap, cataracts, sensorineural deafness, retinopathy, later IDDM (20%)	immunization programmes have reduced the incidence of congenital rubella; all women are screened for immunity at booking
cytomegalovirus	3–4 months	sensorineural deafness, mental handicap (5%)	the most common congenital infection in the UK; most infected children develop normally so a screening programme is not thought necessary
herpes varicella zoster	first trimester	varicella embryopathy, severe scarring of skin, and neurological damage	non-immune pregnant women should be advised to avoid anyone with chickenpox
	5 days before delivery or 2 days after	severe illness as child is not protected by maternal antibodies	exposed children should be given prophylactic zoster immunoglobulin

Fig. 8.12 Congenital infections. (IDDM, insulin-dependent diabetes mellitus.)

- A chromosomal disorder (trisomy 13).
- A single gene disorder (e.g. autosomal dominant polydactyly).
- Unknown aetiology.

Congenital amputations

These occur in 1 in 5000 live births and are due to amniotic bands formed *in utero* by the premature rupture of the amnion, which restricts development of the fetus. Amniotic bands can also cause facial clefts and deformities due to oligohydramnios.

Arthrogryposis

This is a classical example of a multiple malformation and dysmorphic syndrome. It is a heterogeneous group of malformations characterized by stiffness and contractures of the joints of varying severity.

The aetiology can be roughly divided into four groups which are associated with different sub-chromosomal lesions:

- Myopathic (e.g. amyeloplasia).
- Neuropathic (e.g. neural tube defect).
- Connective tissue disorder.
- Extrinsic limitation of fetal movements (e.g. oligohydramnios).

There are flexion contractures of the knee, elbow, and wrist joints, and often the hips are dislocated. Intelligence is usually unaffected. The children are managed with physiotherapy, splints, and surgical correction if unavoidable.

Defects of the CNS

The CNS develops between weeks 3 and 12 of embryonic life. It is an extremely complex and intricate process. Errors can occur at any level. Some of the commoner defects are outlined below.

Neural tube defects (NTDs)

The neural tube is derived from the primitive ectoderm and develops to form the spinal cord and brain. The tube is normally completely closed by the end of week 3 of embryonic development.

The incidence of NTDs of 2–3 in 1000 live births has dropped to 1 in 1000 since the 1970s due to:

- Improved nutrition (dietary supplements of folate around time of conception).

Remember that deformations are correctable, malformations are not correctable.

- Introduction of the routine anomaly ultrasound scan at week 16, providing the opportunity of early termination for severe NTDs.

Defects arise from incomplete closure of the neural tube (Fig. 8.13)

The risk of recurrence in the same family after an affected pregnancy is 1 in 25–33. This can be reduced to 1 in 199 with folate supplements. The recurrence risk for first degree relatives is 1 in 30; 1 in 70 for second degree; and 1 in 150 for third degree.

Holoprosencephaly

This is failure of development of the forebrain and associated midface. About 30% of cases are related to trisomy 13 and there may be a familial element. There is hypotelorism, bilateral cleft lip, and absent philtrum. The most severe cases have a single central eye (cyclops). The child is severely mentally handicapped and does not usually survive more than one month.

Isolated hydrocephalus

An Isolated hydrocephalus refers to enlargement of the ventricular system of the brain in the absence of an NTD. It has an incidence of 0.4 in 1000 live births and results from an imbalance between production and absorption of CSF. Causes include:

- Intracranial haemorrhage.
- Post-infection which has caused CNS scarring.
- Genetic defects.
- Idiopathic.

Brain damage can be avoided by inserting a shunt to allow excess CSF to drain, usually into the peritoneum. Prenatal diagnosis is sometimes possible by serial ultrasound in the second trimester.

Lissencephaly

Lissencephaly means 'smooth brain' and is caused by

defective neuronal migration in months 3–5 of development. It is not detectable on ultrasound and the child often has epilepsy and mental retardation.

Lissencephaly is a feature of the Miller–Dieker syndrome, a microdeletion syndrome of chromosome 17p that can be diagnosed by chromosome analysis.

An isolated lissencephaly has a recurrence risk of 10%.

Macrocephaly and microcephaly

Macrocephaly and microcephaly are defined as head circumferences above the 97th centile and below the 3rd centile, respectively. The causes are listed in Fig. 8.14.

Congenital heart defects

Cardiogenesis occurs between weeks 3 and 8 of embryonic life—a pair of primitive heart tubes fuse and fold to form the four chambers of the heart. Because of the complexity of the process, congenital heart defects are relatively common (7 in 1000 live births).

Congenital heart disease is defined as:

- Cyanotic if the defect causes inadequate oxygenation of the blood due to either underperfusion of the lungs (right-to-left shunt) or inadequate mixing of blood from the pulmonary and systemic circulations.

Neural tube defects		
Part of tube affected	**Defect**	**Features**
rostral end	anencephaly	cranial vault and skin missing; most are stillborn
rostral end	cranium bifidum	defect in cranial vault with protruding meninges with or without brain tissue; surgical correction often successful, especially if brain tissue not involved
caudal end	spina bifida cystica	vertebral arch defect resulting in exposure of spinal cord: meningomyelocoele is the most common and most severe type—the neural tube is completely open so spinal cord lies open and exposed on child's back and severity depends on location (with a small lumbosacral lesion, the child will have good mobility, normal bladder function and intellect; a large thoracolumbar lesion results in paralysed trunk and limbs and hydrocephalus); meningocoele—the neural tube is closed, there is a meningeal sac filled with CSF; neurological problems are rare but there is a risk of complications later in childhood and risk of infection
caudal end	spina bifida occulta	up to 20% of population affected; small defect in vertebral arch; may show tuft of hair over sacrum; risk of cord tethering and bladder problems developing as child grows

Fig. 8.13 Features of neural tube defects.

Fig. 8.14 Causes of microcephaly and macrocephaly.

Causes of microcephaly and macrocephaly	
Microcephaly	**Macrocephaly**
familial small head	familial large head
autosomal recessive condition with severe developmental delay	tall stature
congenital infection (e.g. rubella)	hydrocephalus
	syndrome associated with severe learning difficulties (e.g. Sotos syndrome)
brain damage (e.g. hypoxic ischaemic encephalopathy—hypoxic damage caused by birth asphyxia)	neurofibromatosis
	cerebral tumour
exposure to ionizing radiation during pregnancy	central nervous system storage disorder (e.g. Hurler syndrome)

- Acyanotic if the blood is adequately oxygenated but the defect may cause a left-to-right shunt so the system is very inefficient.

Presentation depends upon severity of the defect. It may be detected on antenatal ultrasound or because of the presence of a heart murmur, cyanosis, heart failure, or shock. Fig. 8.15 describes the common congenital heart diseases. Aetiologically:

- 90% are multifactorial.
- 2% are due to environmental factors.
- 5% are chromosomal disorders .
- 3% are single gene disorders.

Fig. 8.16 lists of some of the factors associated with congenital heart disease.

Fig. 8.15 Common congenital heart diseases.

Common congenital heart diseases		
Lesion	Incidence (livebirths)	Recurrence risk for next pregnancy
ACYANOTIC ventricular septal defect (VSD)	1 in 400	1 in 25
patent ductus arteriosus (PDA)	1 in 830	1 in 33
pulmonary stenosis	1 in 2500	?
atrial septal defect	1 in 1000	1 in 33
coarctation of the aorta	1 in 1600	1 in 50
aortic stenosis	1 in 2000	1 in 50
CYANOTIC tetralogy of Fallot	1 in 1000	1 in 33
transposition of the great arteries	1 in 16 000	1 in 50

Fig. 8.16 Factors associated with congenital heart disease. (ASD, atrial septal defect; PDA, patent ductus arteriosus; VSD, ventricular septal defect.)

Factors associated with congenital heart disease	
Factor	Associated cardiac abnormality
MATERNAL DISORDERS rubella	peripheral pulmonary stenosis, PDA
systemic lupus erythematosus (SLE)	complete heart block (anti-Rho antibody)
alcoholism (fetal alcohol syndrome)	ASD, VSD, tetralogy of Fallot
insulin-dependent diabetes mellitus	incidence increased overall
DRUGS warfarin	pulmonary valve stenosis, PDA
CHROMOSOMAL ABNORMALITY Down syndrome (trisomy 21)	AVSD (40%), VSD (30%), ASD (10%), tetralogy of Fallot (6%)
Edwards' syndrome (trisomy 18)	complex
Patau syndrome (trisomy 13)	complex
Turner syndrome (45X0)	aortic valve stenosis, coarctation of the aorta
chromosome 22 microdeletion	aortic arch anomalies, truncus arteriosus

Gastrointestinal tract defects

These result from defective gastrointestinal organogenesis between weeks 3 and 8 of pregnancy.

Cleft lip and palate

This is due to disordered migration of mesenchymal tissue during development of the face. The occurrence is 1 in 700 live births. It is multifactorial and associated with single gene syndromes, chromosome anomalies, amniotic bands, and maternal drug ingestion (e.g. anticonvulsants, corticosteroids).

There is usually a paramedian cleft in the lip and/or palate, which is unilateral or bilateral. Rarely there is a midline cleft. It requires surgical correction in the first few months of life.

Oesophageal atresia

This is due to failure of communication between the lower end of the oesophagus and stomach, with or without a tracheo-oesophageal fistula (TOF) caused by failure of division of the foregut into respiratory and digestive portions. A TOF can occur without oesophageal atresia and the child aspirates acidic contents, causing scarring of the lungs.

Oesophageal atresia occurs in 1 in 2500 live births. It is multifactorial and associated with:

- Anorectal agenesis.
- Tetralogy of Fallot.
- A familial increased risk of neural tube defects.

There is polyhydramnios during pregnancy and the newborn child chokes and/or vomits on milk.

The defect requires urgent surgical correction to avoid scarring of the lungs.

Anterior abdominal wall defect

There are two types:

- Exomphalos—the persistence of herniation of midgut into the umbilical cord which occurs between weeks 6 and 14 of embryonic life (bowel coated in umbilical cord membranes).
- Gastroschisis—the bowel protrudes through a defect in the anterior abdominal wall (not coated in cord membrane).

The overall occurrence is 1 in 6000 live pregnancies. Exomphalos is associated with trisomy 13 (30%) and congenital heart disease (10%). Gastroschisis has no associated abnormalities.

These defects can be diagnosed on antenatal ultrasound and there is often polyhydramnios. Treatment is by surgical correction as a neonate. A chromosome check should be carried out if there is exomphalos.

Congenital pyloric stenosis

This is due to hypertrophy and hyperplasia of the pyloric muscles causing obstruction to gastric emptying. It is classically seen in the male firstborn child. The occurrence is 1 in 20 male births and 1 in 1000 female births.

Congenital pyloric stenosis presents with projectile vomiting (which is not bile stained), and constipation and dehydration between 4 and 6 weeks of age. (It is not technically congenital as it presents after 2 weeks.) Often there is visible peristalsis and a palpable rubbery tumour below the costal margin on the right-hand side. There is a hypochloraemic alkalosis due to the persistent vomiting. Treatment is surgical division of the muscle fibres.

Duodenal atresia

This results from failure of recanalization of the midgut lumen following the solid stage in week 7. It occurs in 1 in 330 live births and approximately 35% are associated with trisomy 21.

The child presents with bile-stained vomiting. A double air bubble is seen on ultrasound. Urgent surgical correction is required to avoid strangulation.

Hirschsprung's disease

This is due to failure of migration of neural crest cells into the developing hindgut. The affected portion starts at the rectum and the length of gut affected is variable. The occurrence is 1 in 5000–8000 live births; 3♂:1♀. Of these:

- 75% are rectosigmoid.
- 5% affect the entire colon.

The inheritance is multifactorial; however some cases are clearly genetic, associated with the MEN II RET mutation.

Clinically, there is no passage of meconium in the first 48 hours; alternatively, it may present much later in childhood. Abdominal distension develops and there is bile-stained vomiting. Enterocolitis may develop. Surgical removal of the affected portion is indicated.

Imperforate anus

This results from abnormal development of the anorectal septum. It occurs in 1 in 5000 live births and is multifactorial. No anus is visible at birth and there is no passage of meconium. Treatment is by surgical correction.

Kidney and urogenital defects
Intersex conditions
A person with ambiguous genitalia is described as having an intersex condition:

- True hermaphroditism is an extremely rare condition. The person is usually 46XX and has both testicular and ovarian tissue. External genitalia are usually ambiguous.
- A male pseudohermaphrodite is 46XY. The external and internal genitalia are variable. Testicular feminization is a variant of male pseudohermaphroditism in which the karyotype is 46XY with female external genitalia. Testes are present, usually in the inguinal canal. The individual's sexual orientation is female. The condition is caused by insensitivity of the external genitalia to androgens. There is a risk of testicular carcinoma if the testes are not removed surgically.
- Female pseudohermaphroditism is most commonly caused by adrenogenital syndrome. Excess androgens are produced by the fetal suprarenal glands and so the external genitalia are virilized.

Hypospadias
The incidence of hypospadias is 1 in 300 male infants. The urethra opens onto the ventral surface of the shaft of the penis instead of at the tip of the glans. It may result from inadequate production of androgens by the developing fetus.

Defects in renal development
The overall incidence of defects in renal development is 4 in 1000.

Renal agenesis
Renal agenesis affects 1 in 3000 births and the recurrence risk for the parents is 1 in 33. Bilateral renal agenesis results in oligohydramnios, which in turn produces Potter's sequence due to intrauterine compression. (A sequence is a series of abnormalities that can be related to a single primary defect.) The fetus has:

- Large, low-set ears.
- A squashed facies.

- Lung hypoplasia.
- Severe talipes.

Neonatal death is inevitable.

Other causes of severe oligohydramnios can give rise to Potter's sequence, including cystic dysplasia and obstructive uropathy.

Renal hypoplasia and dysplasia
Abnormal renal development can be:

- The result of a single gene defect (e.g. brachio-oto-renal syndrome).
- Part of a dysmorphic syndrome (e.g. Noonan's syndrome, Turner's syndrome).

The majority are unexplained and have a low recurrence risk. There is a risk of renal failure and inadvertent removal of abnormal kidneys during abdominal surgery!

Infantile polycystic syndrome
This is a rare autosomal recessive condition resulting in cysts in the liver, kidneys, and pancreas. These interfere with function, leading to death in early childhood.

Multiple malformations and dysmorphic syndromes
Multiple malformations are present in 0.7% of neonates. A minority of these show patterns that allow them to be identified as one of the 2000 dysmorphic syndromes that have been described. The genetic bases of the dysmorphic syndromes covered in this section have not yet been identified. Other dysmorphic syndromes have already been described earlier in this section.

Beckwith–Wiedemann syndrome
This has an incidence of 1 in 3700 live births. There is paternal duplication of 11p15 and some are autosomal dominant with variable expression. Complications include:

- Macroglossia.
- Anterior abdominal wall defect.
- High birth weight.
- Hemihypertrophy.

Approximately 10% develop neoplasia—Wilms' tumour, hepatoblastoma, rhabdomyosarcoma, or adrenal cortical carcinoma. Serial ultrasound is indicated for the first three years of life to detect cancers.

CHARGE association

CHARGE is a sporadic non-random association of:

- **C**oloboma.
- **H**eart defects.
- Cho**A**nal atresia.
- **R**etarded growth.
- **G**enital abnormalities.
- Abnormal **E**ars.

This association is a non-random combination of two or more defects that are not due to the same embryological defect.

DiGeorge syndrome

This is actually a sequence, as defects relate to a single developmental abnormality. There is a sporadic microdeletion at 22q11. Defects result from abnormal development of branchial arch 4 and pharyngeal pouches 3 and 4.

Clinical features include:

- Neonatal seizures secondary to hypoparathyroidism.
- Recurrent infections secondary to athymia.
- Failure to thrive.
- Aortic arch anomalies.
- Dysmorphic face with hypertelorism, down-slanting palpebral fissures, and fish-like mouth.

The severity of the defects varies.

Noonan's syndrome

This has an incidence of 1 in 2000 and it is autosomal dominant in some families. The majority of the cases are sporadic. Features include:

- Characteristic facies (low-set ears and down-slanting eyes).
- Mild learning difficulties.
- Short webbed neck with trident hair line.
- Short stature.
- Congenital heart disease (especially pulmonary stenosis, ASD).

VATER association

VATER association involves:

- **V**ertebral defects.
- **A**nal atresia.
- **T**racheo-oesophageal fistula.
- **RE**nal defects.
- **R**adial limb defects.

(Congenital heart disease, and a single umbilical artery are also associated).

Williams syndrome

This has an incidence of 1 in 20 000. There is deletion in 7q11.23 and this may be sporadic or autosomal dominant. Features include:

- Mental retardation.
- Gregarious personality.
- Infantile hypocalcaemia.
- Characteristic facies with a broad forehead, big mouth, prominent ear lobes, and micrognathia.

- What is the difference between a congenital deformation and a congenital malformation?
- Outline the five major maternal infections that cause congenital malformations.
- What is a neural tube defect? What sorts of congenital malformations can they cause?
- List the major cyanotic and acyanotic congenital heart defects. What are the major associated risk factors?
- Write short notes on congenital gastrointestinal tract defects—cleft lip and palate, oesophageal atresia, anterior abdominal wall defect, congenital pyloric stenosis, duodenal atresia, Hirschsprung's disease, imperforate anus.
- What is meant by hermaphroditism? Differentiate between true and pseudohermaphroditism.
- What is Potter's sequence?
- Give some examples of dysmorphic syndromes.

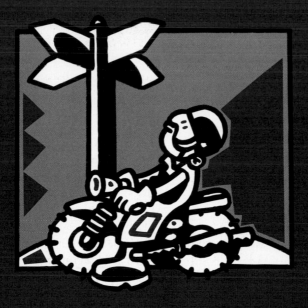

SELF-ASSESSMENT

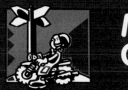
Indicate whether each answer is true or false.

1. Concerning the cell:

(a) Its size is limited by diffusion.
(b) Its size is limited by osmosis.
(c) If prokaryotic, it has a nucleus.
(d) If eukaryotic, it undergoes binary reproduction.
(e) Prokaryotes are larger than eukaryotes.

2. Concerning organelles:

(a) Mitochondria have a phospholipid bilayer.
(b) The plasma membrane is an organelle.
(c) Smooth endoplasmic reticulum makes polypeptides.
(d) Peroxisomes are larger than lysosomes.
(e) Mitochondria can reproduce independently.

3. Concerning amino acids:

(a) D-isomers are found in humans.
(b) Essential amino acids are synthesized in humans.
(c) Glycine is the smallest amino acid.
(d) Cysteine can form disulphide bridges.
(e) The carboxyl group gives acidic properties.

4. In protein structure:

(a) The quaternary structure is the final three-dimensional shape.
(b) The primary structure determines the three-dimensional shape.
(c) Cysteine is usually found at α helix bends.
(d) The polypeptide bond is very flexible.
(e) Hydrophobic bond energy is obtained from water displacement.

5. Concerning protein function:

(a) Full activity is seen in the tertiary structure.
(b) Shaking can destroy function.
(c) Cofactors are proteins required for protein function.
(d) A prosthetic group is conjugated to a protein.
(e) Proteins can function as storage molecules.

6. Concerning enzymes:

(a) If extracellular they are made outside the cell.
(b) Isoenzymes have the same structure, but catalyse different reactions.
(c) They are consumed by the reactions they catalyse.
(d) Lyases break down covalent carbon bonds.
(e) They can work in both directions of the reaction.

7. In enzyme kinetics:

(a) The initial velocity is the reaction rate.
(b) First order kinetics are seen by increasing enzyme concentration.
(c) Low substrate concentration is seen in zero order kinetics.
(d) A low K_m is seen with high enzyme substrate affinity.
(e) Competitive inhibitors increase the K_m.

8. In the fluid mosaic model:

(a) The membrane is 6–10 nm wide.
(b) Cholesterol is the major lipid.
(c) Phospholipid structure has a glycerol with three fatty acid groups attached.
(d) Integral proteins are very hydrophobic.
(e) Non-ionic detergents have poor solubilizing properties.

9. Properties of membranes include:

(a) Greater permeability to ionic and polar compounds than lipid-soluble compounds.
(b) Cholesterol increases fluidity at body temperature.
(c) Uneven distribution of membrane lipids.
(d) Increasing transition temperature with the chain length of membrane fatty acids.
(e) Decreasing transition temperature with degree of saturation of membrane fatty acids.

10. Concerning ionic distributions across the membrane:

(a) There are more amino acids inside the cell.
(b) There is more sodium outside the cell.
(c) A hypotonic intracellular solution causes water to move into the cell.
(d) A hypotonic extracellular solution causes water to move into the cell.
(e) The sodium pump maintains an equilibrium across the cell membrane.

11. In membrane transport:

(a) Ionic channels are non-specific.
(b) Facilitated diffusion requires specific carrier proteins.
(c) Carrier proteins can be linked to an energy source.
(d) Facilitated diffusion follows Fick's law of diffusion.
(e) Gated ion channels transport molecules by passive diffusion.

12. In membrane potential:

(a) The resting potential is negative inside with respect to the outside.
(b) Proteins are cations, so attract diffusible anions.
(c) The compartment volumes need to be fixed for the Gibbs–Donnan effect.
(d) The Gibbs–Donnan effect causes the cell membrane potential.
(e) In depolarization the membrane potential becomes more negative inside relative to the outside.

13. Transmembrane signalling:

(a) Is the path by which all cells are directed to divide and differentiate.
(b) May malfunction along its pathway and cause carcinoma.
(c) Involves many more second messengers than receptors.
(d) Involves oncogenes as part of the signalling pathway.
(e) Has a ligand as the first receptor.

14. Concerning actin:

(a) It gives phagocytes motility.
(b) It forms the structure of cilia.
(c) It forms the structure of microvilli.
(d) Actin-binding proteins are called microfilament accessory proteins.
(e) Colchicine causes its depolymerization.

15. Concerning microtubules:

(a) They are more stable than intermediate filaments.
(b) An example is cytokeratin.
(c) They are formed of dimeric structural units.
(d) They are found in immature erythrocytes.
(e) Kinesins, which are associated proteins, move in an antegrade direction.

16. Concerning lysosomes:

(a) They are found in erythrocytes.
(b) Lysozyme is normally found inside.
(c) Phagocytosis is a form of endocytosis.
(d) Heterophagy is digestion of material of intracellular origin.
(e) Progressive neurological degeneration is a feature of lysosmal storage diseases.

17. Concerning cell junctions:

(a) An adhesion belt can attach cells to the matrix.
(b) Desmosomes are made of intermediate filaments.
(c) Adhesion belts are held together by cadherins.
(d) Gap junctions can be gated.
(e) Electrical coupling can occur via gap junctions.

18. Concerning adhesion molecules:

(a) The immunoglobulin family have calcium-dependent adhesion.
(b) MAC1 is an integrin.
(c) Selectins have a lectin domain.
(d) Lectin domains recognize oligosaccharides on neutrophils.
(e) Cadherins can undergo homophilic binding.

19. Concerning inheritance patterns:

(a) O is the symbol for a female in pedigree charts.
(b) Sex chromosomes are autosomes.
(c) Penetrance is defined as a range of phenotypes produced by a single gene.
(d) Phenotype is determined by genotype and environment.
(e) ∅ is the symbol for a deceased female in pedigree charts.

20. In X-linked recessive inheritance:

(a) An affected male will have daughters who are all carriers.
(b) Affected males may have an affected father.
(c) Haemophilia is an example.
(d) Thalassaemia is an example.
(e) Women may be affected if there is skewed lyonization.

21. In single gene disorder mutations:

(a) A purine to purine substitution is called a transversion.
(b) A splice site substitution causes a quantitative change in the protein.
(c) Increasing paternal age increases dominant mutations.
(d) Dystrophin mutations are normally large.
(e) Point mutations may not cause any effect.

22. In Down syndrome:

(a) Diagnosis can be achieved by screening pregnancies.
(b) Alzheimer's disease is seen in all individuals by 40 years of age.
(c) Its occurrence is 1 in 650 live births.
(d) It can be diagnosed by appearance.
(e) It is commonly associated with meconium ileus.

23. In Turner's syndrome:

(a) IQ is normal.
(b) The cause is a mutation affecting the long arm of X.
(c) It is commonly associated with congenital heart disease.
(d) It is commonly detected on ultrasound.
(e) It is seen in 1 in 2500 liveborn males.

24. In cystic fibrosis:

(a) The gene is located on chromosome 7.
(b) Population screening identifies many cases.
(c) $1/22$ of the British population are carriers.
(d) Death can be due to heat prostration.
(e) 68% are due to a mutation at codon 508.

25. In Duchenne muscular dystrophy:

(a) $2/3$ are new mutations.
(b) Dystrophin is the largest known gene.
(c) Creatinine is raised.
(d) Decreased intracellular calcium causes wasting.
(e) Wasting is symmetrical.

26. Concerning the nucleus:

(a) The diameter is generally about 5 μm.
(b) Euchromatin is not actively expressed.
(c) Barr bodies are seen in female cells.
(d) Nucleoli are very active in the synthesis of messenger RNA (mRNA).
(e) All cells in the human body have nuclei.

27. The cell cycle:

(a) Is a continuous process that is unaffected by the surrounding environment.
(b) Does not occur in malignant cells.
(c) Is controlled directly by phosphorylation of regulatory proteins.
(d) Has intrinsic control exerted by hormones.
(e) Has extrinsic control exerted by cyclins.

28. Concerning cell replication:

(a) A polyploid cell contains more than one set of chromosomes.
(b) Cyclin A is the cyclin involved in the initiation of mitosis.
(c) Haploid cells contain two full sets of chromosomes.
(d) Transfer of genetic information between homologous chromosomes occurs during prophase I of meiosis.
(e) Mitotic cell division always produces genetically identical daughter cells.

29. Concerning purines and pyrimidines:

(a) They are vital components of nucleotides but not nucleosides.
(b) In humans, they are synthesized entirely *de novo*.
(c) Adenine and cytosine are both examples of purines.
(d) Guanine and thymine are both examples of pyrimidines.
(e) They are associated with a pentose sugar and a phosphate group to form nucleotides.

30. Concerning nucleic acids:

(a) Viruses do not contain nucleic acids.
(b) In DNA, cytosine pairs with guanine.
(c) In RNA, adenine pairs with thymine.
(d) All RNA forms a double helix under physiological conditions.
(e) They are polymers of nucleotides.

31. Within the nucleus:

(a) Chromatin consists of DNA and RNA only.
(b) Histone proteins are negatively charged.
(c) The nucleosome core protein consists of eight histone subunits.
(d) H1 histone is not found in the core protein.
(e) HNPCC: (hereditary non-polyposis coli) is caused by a defect in excision repair.

32. Okasaki fragments:

(a) Are generated from the lag strand of DNA.
(b) Occur in the eukaryotic DNA replication process only.
(c) Are manufactured on the lead strand of parent DNA.
(d) Are joined together by a DNA gyrase.
(e) Reflect the fact that DNA polymerases can read 3'–5' only.

33. Concerning DNA replication:

(a) Prokaryotic nuclei contain a single species of DNA polymerase.
(b) Replication is initiated at a single origin in prokaryotes, but multiple origins in eukaryotics.
(c) Occurs during the M1 phase of the cell cycle.
(d) The process is conservative replication.
(e) The copy error rate for mammalian polymerases is one in 10^8–10^{10} base pairs.

34. Concerning the genetic code:

(a) Genetic code refers to the manner in which RNA codes for amino acids.
(b) It displays degeneracy.
(c) mRNA can be polycistronic in eukaryotes.
(d) Codons are formed from triplets of three amino acids.
(e) The triplet of adenine, uracil + guanine (AUG) codes for methionine.

35. The wobble hypothesis.

(a) Accounts for unexpected base pair associations between mRNA and transfer RNA (tRNA).
(b) Applies to non-Watson-Crick base pairing between the mRNA codon and first base on tRNA.
(c) Increases with tRNA base modification.
(d) A uracil base on the tRNA will pair with either guanine or adenine on the mRNA.
(e) Differs in mitochondria.

36. Concerning DNA transcription:

(a) Prokaryotic cells contain a single species of RNA polymerase.
(b) In eukaryotes, it can occur in the cytoplasm.
(c) DNA is used as a template for the synthesis of RNA.
(d) Transcription termination by hairpin formation is a feature of eukaryotic cells.
(e) The Shine–Dalgarno sequence is involved in prokaryotic transcription initiation.

37. Concerning post-transcriptional modification:

(a) This is sometimes not necessary in prokaryotes.
(b) It usually involves the addition of a poly-A tail in eukaryotic transcripts.
(c) Splicing involves the removal of exons from the heterogeneous nuclear RNA (hnRNA).
(d) Snurps consist entirely of RNA.
(e) The eukaryotic 5' methyl cap protects the transcript from enzymatic degradation.

38. Concerning translation:

(a) This is the manufacture of proteins directly from DNA.
(b) Triplets of nucleotides code for each amino acid.
(c) It occurs on the endoplasmic reticulum of eukaryotic cells.
(d) The Shine–Dalgarno sequence is involved in eukaryotic translation initiation.
(e) It can be targeted by antimicrobial agents because prokaryotic and eukaryotic ribosomes are different.

39. Post-translational modification includes:

(a) The addition of a signal peptide to proteins bound for export.
(b) Carboxylation of procollagen to form collagen.
(c) Processes that take place in the cytoplasm.
(d) Cleavage of proinsulin to produce insulin.
(e) Some processes that occur as the protein is being translated.

40. Concerning HIV infection:

(a) The virus is a double stranded RNA virus.
(b) The virus replicates in the cytoplasm of its host.
(c) It is characterized by the progressive destruction of the host's bone marrow.
(d) It targets CD8+ T cells.
(e) Combination therapy is considered to be more effective than monotherapy.

41. Concerning bacteria:

(a) They contain a nuclear membrane.
(b) Cell wall synthesis can be targeted by sulphonamides.
(c) Penicillin can be used in the treatment of meningococcal meningitis.
(d) They have a sexual form of reproduction called conjugation.
(e) Transduction can only occur in the absence of viruses.

42. Bayes' theorem:

(a) Can be used to calculate allele frequencies in a population.
(b) Uses calculations based on mendelian genetics.
(c) Can be used to assess a couple's risk of having an affected child.
(d) Predicts absolute risk.
(e) Can be applied to calculate risk using existing information.

43. In genetic counselling:

(a) Paternity testing can be accurately carried out using DNA fingerprinting.
(b) Consanguinity can cause an increased frequency of autosomal recessive conditions.
(c) An accurate diagnosis is not always necessary.
(d) In the UK it is legal to marry your cousin.
(e) An accurate family history is of paramount importance.

44. Concerning the Hardy–Weinberg equation:

(a) It applies only if a population is in equilibrium.
(b) It can be used to calculate allele frequencies in a population.
(c) For an autosomal recessive condition, incidence is calculated as q^2.
(d) For an autosomal dominant condition, disease frequency is approximately equal to frequency of homozygotes.
(e) It will not apply if there is a mass migration.

45. Concerning population screening:

(a) It aims to detect people with a disease.
(b) Early diagnosis must be advantageous.
(c) The Guthrie test is used to detect phenylketonuria only.
(d) A routine anomalies ultrasound scan is performed at 16–18 weeks of pregnancy.
(e) The Triple test tests for maternal serum α-fetoprotein, β-human gonadotrophic hormone, and progesterone.

46. Concerning neural tube defects:

(a) They are examples of congenital deformations.
(b) Defects arise from incomplete closure of the neural tube.
(c) Holoprosencephaly is associated with trisomy 17.
(d) A myelomeningocoele is a type of spina bifida.
(e) Cranium bifidum is never compatible with life.

47. Ataxia telangiectasia:

(a) Is caused by a defect in excision repair.
(b) Is caused by a defect in mismatch repair.
(c) Can be diagnosed by telangiectasia in the eyes.
(d) Carries a very high risk of colon cancer.
(e) Is associated with myeloproliferative disease.

48. Features of fragile X syndrome include:

(a) Usually male.
(b) Big ears.
(c) Usually severe learning difficulties.
(d) Father to son transmission.
(e) Cytosine, guanine, guanine (CGG) triplet repeat expansion.

49. Concerning congenital malformations:

(a) Most are caused by an underlying chromosomal abnormality.
(b) They are caused by an error of development.
(c) 5% of congenital heart disease is due to a chromosomal defect.
(d) Macrocephaly and microcephaly refer to brain size.
(e) Congenital renal agenesis results in Williams syndrome.

50. Congenital rubella:

(a) Is most likely to occur if the mother has a primary infection at 3–4 months of pregnancy.
(b) Causes cataracts.
(c) Causes severe learning difficulties.
(d) Is increasing in incidence.
(e) Is associated with insulin-dependent diabetes mellitus.

Short-answer Questions

1. List five differences between prokaryotic and eukaryotic cells.

2. Describe the four levels of protein organization.

3. Draw a diagram to show the fluid mosaic model of the cell membrane.

4. Show the structure of a typical active transporter.

5. What is the difference between endocrine, autocrine, and paracrine signalling?

6. What is the structure of cilia?

7. Define and give examples of gene penetrance and expressivity.

8. Explain what anticipation is and where it is seen, giving three examples.

9. What is Knudson's two-hit hypothesis?

10. What symptoms and signs are seen in mucopolysaccharidoses?

11. What is a nucleosome and what are the proteins present in this structure?

12. Describe what is meant by a vector and outline the use of vectors in DNA technology.

13. List the biological components necessary for translation of messenger RNA (mRNA) to a protein in a prokaryotic cell.

14. Briefly describe how DNA fragments produced by restriction enzyme digestion by EcoR1 can be separated and visualized.

15. Draw a simple pedigree of three generations of a family to illustrate the transmission of an X-linked recessive disorder.

16. Draw a diagram to illustrate the important features of a transfer RNA (tRNA) molecule.

17. State three ways by which bacteria acquire DNA from other bacteria in nature and indicate one clinically important consequence of these processes.

18. Indicate how the following three listed antibiotics exert their antibacterial effects:
    (a) Tetracycline.
    (b) Chloramphenicol.
    (c) Streptomycin.

19. Draw a diagram of the cell cycle with the following marked clearly upon it: S, M, G_1, and G_2 phases. Indicate the points in the cycle at which growth factors, M-phase promoting factor (MPF), and S-phase activating factor exert their influence and where cells can enter the quiescent state (G_0).

20. How are amino acids 'activated' in the translation stage of protein synthesis?

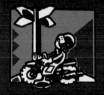

Essay Questions

1. What effects do different inhibitors have on reaction rate in enzyme kinetics?

2. Explain what is meant by imprinting, with examples.

3. What factors affect mutation type and frequency?

4. Explain what is meant by mitochondrial inheritance and list typical clinical features with examples.

5. Explain receptor-mediated endocytosis.

6. Describe the principles of the polymerase chain reaction and discuss its uses in prenatal diagnosis.

7. Give an outline of the structure of DNA, paying particular attention to the role played by hydrogen bonds. How do the structural defects in DNA associated with the disease xeroderma pigmentosum arise?

8. Give an account of the post-transcriptional events that precede the transport of messenger RNA (mRNA) from the nucleus to the cytoplasm.

9. Describe the chief events of mitosis and show how these differ from meiosis.

10. Describe the events associated with the replication of DNA in prokaryotic cells. Indicate how this process differs in eukaryotic cells.

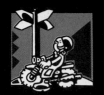

MCQ Answers

1. (a)T, (b)F, (c)F, (d)F, (e)F
2. (a)T, (b)T, (c)F, (d)F, (e)T
3. (a)F, (b)F, (c)T, (d)T, (e)T
4. (a)F, (b)T, (c)F, (d)F, (e)T
5. (a)F, (b)T, (c)F, (d)T, (e)T
6. (a)F, (b)F, (c)F, (d)T, (e)T
7. (a)T, (b) T, (c)F, (d)T, (e)T
8. (a)T, (b)F, (c)F, (d)T, (e)T
9. (a)F, (b)F, (c)T, (d)T, (e)F
10. (a)T, (b)F, (c)F, (d)T, (e)F
11. (a)F, (b)T, (c)T, (d)F, (e)T
12. (a)T, (b)F, (c)T, (d)F, (e)T
13. (a)T, (b)T, (c)F, (d)T, (e)T
14. (a)T, (b)F, (c)T, (d)T, (e)F
15. (a)F, (b)F, (c)T, (d)T, (e)T
16. (a)F, (b)F, (c)F, (d)F, (e)T
17. (a)F, (b)T, (c)T, (d)T, (e)T
18. (a)F, (b)T, (c)T, (d)T, (e)T
19. (a)F, (b)F, (c)F, (d)T, (e)T
20. (a)T, (b)F, (c)T, (d)F, (e)T
21. (a)F, (b)F, (c)T, (d)T, (e)T
22. (a)F, (b)T, (c)T, (d)F, (e)F
23. (a)T, (b)F, (c)T, (d)F, (e)F
24. (a)T, (b)F, (c)T, (d)T, (e)T
25. (a)F, (b)T, (c)F, (d)F, (e)T

26. (a)T, (b)F, (c)T, (d)F, (e)F
27. (a)F, (b)F, (c)T, (d)F, (e)F
28. (a)F, (b)F, (c)F, (d)T, (e)F
29. (a)F, (b)F, (c)F, (d)F, (e)T
30. (a)F, (b)T, (c)F, (d)F, (e)T
31. (a)F, (b)F, (c)T, (d)T, (e)F
32. (a)T, (b)F, (c)F, (d)F, (e)T
33. (a)F, (b)T, (c)F, (d)F, (e)T
34. (a)T, (b)T, (c)F, (d)F, (e)T
35. (a)T, (b)F, (c)T, (d)F, (e)T
36. (a)T, (b)F, (c)T, (d)F, (e)F
37. (a)T, (b)T, (c)T, (d)F, (e)T
38. (a)F, (b)T, (c)T, (d)F, (e)T
39. (a)F, (b)F, (c)T, (d)T, (e)T
40. (a)F, (b)F, (c)F, (d)F, (e)T
41. (a)F, (b)F, (c)T, (d)T, (e)F
42. (a)F, (b)T, (c)T, (d)F, (e)T
43. (a)T, (b)T, (c)F, (d)T, (e)T
44. (a)T, (b)T, (c)T, (d)F, (e)T
45. (a)F, (b)T, (c)F, (d)T, (e)F
46. (a)F, (b)T, (c)F, (d)T, (e)F
47. (a)T, (b)F, (c)T, (d)F, (e)T,
48. (a)T, (b)T, (c)F, (d)F, (e)T
49. (a)F, (b)T, (c)T, (d)F, (e)F
50. (a)T, (b)T, (c)T, (d)F, (e)T

1. See Fig. 1.

2. Protein organization can be divided into:
   - Primary structure—the linear amino acid polypeptide sequence determined by DNA.
   - Secondary structure—the coiling of local polypeptide regions with the formation of maximum hydrogen bonds and side chain repulsion (e.g. α helices and β pleated sheets).
   - Tertiary structure—side chain interaction causing folding into the unique three-dimensional polypeptide shape (e.g. haemoglobin β chain).
   - Quaternary structure—polypeptide chains interact to form a protein that is biologically active (e.g. four chains form haemoglobin around a prosthetic haem group).

3. See Fig. 3.1.

4. Use sodium pump as the example—tetramer of two glycosylated α units and two non-glycosylated β units. The α subunit is catalytic, binding sodium and adenosine triphosphate (ATP) intracellularly and potassium extracellularly (see Fig. 3.13).

5. See Fig. 3.20.

6. Cilia are formed from microtubules in a 9+2 arrangement, with a basal body in a 9-triplet arrangement (Fig. 4.6). Dynein arms connect adjacent microtubule pairs, and their sliding mechanism enables the cilia to bend.

7. Penetrance means that a gene defect is not expressed in all individuals with the mutation. It is expressed as the proportion of individuals with the mutation (gene defect) that have symptoms (e.g. Huntington's disease has 100% penetrance, so all individuals with the gene have symptoms). Expressivity is a range of phenotypes produced by a single gene defect (e.g. tuberous sclerosis can range from asymptomatic to fatal).

8. Anticipation means the age of onset decreases and/or severity of a disease increases as a gene is passed through generations. It is seen in trinucleotide repeat disorders such as myotonic dystrophy, fragile X syndrome, Huntington's disease, or any other trinucleotide repeat disorder.

9. Knudson's two-hit hypothesis is the mechanism by which tumour suppressor gene function is lost (see Fig. 6.21).

10. Symptoms and signs of mucopolysaccharidoses are progressive neurological degeneration, hepatosplenomegaly, skeletal dysplasia, short stature, bone pain, coarse facies, ocular cherry red spots, and corneal clouding.

11. A nucleosome is a complex of DNA wrapped around a protein complex called the core protein particle. It forms the first level of DNA packaging in the nucleus. Histone proteins are present in the structure. Eight histones complex to form the core protein particle, which has the composition: $(H2A)_2(H2B)_2(H3)_2(H4)_2$. H1 histone lies over the DNA, separate from the core protein particle.

12. A vector is a self-replicating unit that can be used to generate DNA clones. It must contain an origin of replication so that it can replicate in a host cell. Fragments of DNA to be cloned are ligated into the vector. The ligated product can be transfected into a host cell, which will generate identical copies of the target DNA. Vectors often contain a selectable marker such as an antibiotic resistance gene.

Prokaryotic compared with eukaryotic cells	
Prokaryotic	**Eukaryotic**
1–10 μm	10–100 μm
no nucleus	nucleus
no membrane-bound organelles	organelles
binary reproduction	mitotic reproduction
no specialization	specialization into tissues and organs

Fig. 1 Prokaryotic versus eukaryotic cells.

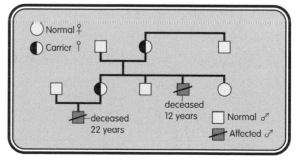

Fig. 2 Simple pedigree of three generations of a family to illustrate the transmission of an X-linked recessive disorder. (Note the absence of male–male transmission because affected males generally die before reproductive age.)

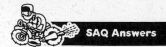

13. Messenger RNA (mRNA), transfer RNA (tRNA), ribosome, guanosine triphosphate (GTP), initiation factors, elongation factors.

14. The fragments can be separated by gel electrophoresis. In this process, the DNA is placed into wells at the top of a piece of polyacrylamide gel. A potential difference is applied to the gel and since DNA is negatively charged it migrates towards the positive electrode. The smaller the DNA fragment, the more mobile it is, so it travels further towards the anode. This can be used to assess DNA fragment size. The fragment sizes can be visualized by soaking the gel in ethidium bromide and viewing it under ultraviolet light.

15. See Fig. 2. The carrier ♀ passes the mutation on to her daughter on an X chromosome. Neither woman is severely affected as they have normal copies of the gene on their other X chromosome. The daughter passes the mutation onto her son on an X chromosome. He inherits a Y chromosome from his father and consequently does not have a normal copy of the gene; hence the resultant disease.

16. See Fig. 5.14. Your diagram should have a clover-leaf structure and five arms: dihydrouridine arm on the left; TψC arm on the right; acceptor arm (with amino acid attached to CCA group at 3′ teminus) pointing up; and anticodon arm (with anticodon on the base) pointing downwards. The variable arm should be between the anticodon and TψC arms—this bit is for honours students!

17. Bacteria acquire DNA through:
    - Transformation.
    - Transduction.
    - Conjugation.

    Genetic transfer is important in the development of antibiotic-resistant pathogens.

18. (a) Tetracycline inhibits prokaryotic protein synthesis by preventing aminoacyl-tRNA binding to the 30 S ribosomal subunit.
    (b) Chloramphenicol inhibits prokaryotic protein synthesis by inhibiting peptidyl transferase.
    (c) Streptomycin inhibits prokaryotic protein synthesis by binding to the 30 S ribosomal subunit, causing mRNA misreading and preventing chain initiation/elongation.

19. See top part of Fig. 5.4.

20. Amino acids are activated during combination with IRNA in a reaction catalyzed by a specific aminoacyl transferase. This incorporates a 'high-energy' ester bond between the aminoacyl group and the 3′ CCA group of the tRNA. Energy released from hydrolysis of this bond drives the peptide bond formation step of chain elongation:

$$\text{Amino acid} + \text{tRNA} \xrightarrow{\text{aminoacyl transferase}} \text{Aminoacyl-tRNA}$$

Index

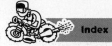

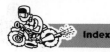

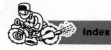

lysine, 13, 14
lysophospholipids, 31
lysosomal storage diseases, 54–6
lysosomes, 7, 8, 54–6
    definition, 54
    functions, 54

M

MAC1, 62
macrocephaly, 146, 172
macro-orchidism, 150
major histocompatibility complex (MHC) antigens, 58, 122
mannose-6-phosphate, 54
MAP1C, 51, 52
Marfan syndrome, 65, 146, 149, 159
maternal serum screening, 131, 132–3
mating, non-random, 121
Maxam–Gilbert method of DNA sequencing, 135, 138
medical history, past, 144
meiosis, 71, 72–3
melanoma, malignant, 147
MELAS syndrome, 165
membrane
    basement, 63
    cell, 29–47
    components, 29–32
    fluidity, 32–3
    fluid mosaic model, 29
    ion distribution across, 34–5
    mobility of components, 33
    permeability, 33
    plasma, 5
    pores, 35, 36
    properties, 32–3
    proteins see proteins, membrane
    receptors, 41–7
    recycling, 8
    semipermeable, 34, 38
    structure, 29–33
    transport see transport, transmembrane
membrane potential, 37, 38–41
    definition, 38
    maintenance, 38–40
    potassium ion effect, 40
    resting, 40
membranous organelles, 5–8
Mendelian inheritance, 111–13, 116
mental retardation, 122, 148
MERAF syndrome, 165
messenger RNA (mRNA), 5, 76, 91
    addition of 5' cap, 88–9
    synthesis, 87, 88
metabolic myopathies, 148

metabotropic receptors, 44–6
metaphase, 71, 72
methicillin-resistant *Staphylococcus aureus* (MRSA), 104
methionine, 13
micelle formation, 32
Michaelis constant (K_m), 25, 26
Michaelis–Menten graph, 25
microcephaly, 146, 172
microfilament accessory proteins, 49–50
microfilaments, 9, 49
microphthalmos, 147
microtubule associated proteins (MAPs), 51
microtubule organizing centre (MTOC), 78
microtubules, 9, 50–1
microvilli, 5, 9, 52, 53
migration, 121
Miller–Dieker syndrome, 172
minisatellite loci, 130, 131
mitochondria, 6
    antibiotic actions, 98–9
    DNA, 93, 94
    RNA synthesis, 88
mitochondrial inheritance, 114–15, 163–5
mitosis, 68, 69, 71–2
mitosis promoting factor (MPF), 69–70
mitotic spindle, 53
moles, 34
mongoloid slant, 146
monosomy X see Turner's syndrome
mosaicism, 113–14
    germline, 114
    somatic, 114
motility, cell, 49–53
motor skills
    fine, 145
    gross, 145
M phase, 69
mucopolysaccharidoses, 150, 164
multiple endocrine neoplasia (MEN), 166–7
muscle cells (fibres), 4
    contraction, 52
    membrane potentials, 40, 41
muscular dystrophies, 148, 163
mutagenesis, site-directed, 138–40
mutagens, chemical, 79
mutations, 79, 120
    frequency, 121
    point, 121
    screening techniques, 135–8
myoglobin, 18
myosin, 20, 51
myotonic dystrophy (MD), 122, 156, 157
    clinical features, 146, 148, 157, 158

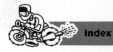